VALERIAN

The Relaxing and Sleep Herb

by Christopher Hobbs

Botanica Press, Capitola, CA

Look for other books available from
Botanica Press by **Christopher Hobbs**

The Herbs and Health Series:

Foundations of Health - The Liver and Digestion Herbal
Echinacea! The Immune Herb
Ginkgo, Elixir of Youth
Milk Thistle: The Liver Herb
Vitex: The Women's Herb
Usnea: The Herbal Antibiotic
Medicinal Mushrooms
Natural Liver Therapy
Handbook for Herbal Healing
Kombucha Manchurian Tea Mushroom

Copyright © August, 1993
by Christopher Hobbs
3rd printing, October, 1995

Michael Miovic, *editor*
Beth Baugh, *supervising editor*
Anatomy illustration © July 1993 by Marni Fylling
Plectritis congesta illustration © July 1993 by D.D. Dowden
Cover Photo © 1993 by Steven Foster

Botanica Press
10226 Empire Grade
Santa Cruz, CA 95060

Our Commitment

We at Botanica Press are dedicated in our personal and professional lives to environmental awareness. We are strongly committed to recycling, and we gladly contribute a portion of our profits to the Nature Conservancy and other conservation groups. This book is printed on recycled paper with a minimum of 10% post-consumer waste, and the entire text is printed using soy-based ink.

 This book is printed on recycled paper.

Author's Disclaimer

The information in this book is intended for educational purposes, not as a prescription for any specific ailment. If you have a serious illness, the author recommends consulting a qualified holistic health practitioner or medical doctor.

TABLE OF CONTENTS

INTRODUCTION

Down through the ages valerian has been and continues to be one of the most popular and widely used medicinal herbs. It is an herbal sedative that is as famous in natural medicine as Valium is in the allopathic system of medicine. That relaxants and sedatives—herbal or otherwise—are needed in today's hectic world is reflected in the following statistics:

- 5% of all people in industrialized countries are affected by anxiety
- 10% of people in the United States take benzodiazepines such as Librium, Valium, or Xanax
- 15% of the American adult population (35 million people) have hypertension
- 33% of the U.S. population consider chronic insomnia a problem

So if you or someone you know is suffering from any sort of nervous disorder, read on. Valerian is a safe and effective natural alternative to the harsh and potentially toxic synthetic sedatives many people commonly take. And not only is valerian's medicinal value confirmed by centuries of popular use, but recently it has also been demonstrated in well-designed scientific studies.

The aim of this book is to present valuable information about valerian in an accessible format. The first half of the book is dedicated to lay readers. I have made every attempt to explain the latest scientific findings on valerian in simple, understandable terms. I have also provided plenty of practical information about:

- What ailments and conditions valerian is good for
- How much valerian to take and for how long
- What the best valerian products are and how to take them

The second half of this book (the appendix) is intended for more technically-minded readers. Here I present detailed, scientific information on the botany, chemistry, pharmacology, and cultivation of valerian. Please note that the information on cultivation may be of interest not only to scientists, but also to those who are interested in growing, processing, or preparing their own valerian medicines. Many herbalists feel that a personal connection with an herb increases its healing power.

In any case, whether you believe in the traditional wisdom concerning valerian, or the modern research, or *both*, you should find a wealth of useful information in this book.

SEDATIVE AND SLEEP-PROMOTING DRUGS

A sedative is a drug that decreases activity in the central nervous system (brain and spinal cord). The degree of sedation a person experiences can range from mild to strong (i.e., sleep), depending on the strength and amount of sedative taken. Doctors generally use sedatives for the following (after Wilson et al., 1977):

1. Sudden, limited, stressful situations involving great emotional strain (for example, a trip to the dentist)
2. Chronic tension states created by disease or sociologic factors (such as urban crime, family problems, or job stress)
3. Hypertension (high blood pressure)
4. Potentiation of analgesic (pain-relieving) drugs
5. Control of convulsions (as in epilepsy)
6. Adjuncts to anesthesia
7. Psychiatric uses (anxiety, neurosis, mania, etc.)
8. Insomnia

Sedatives have been used since ancient times. The first sedative was probably alcohol made from fermented grains (Wilson et al., 1977). The opium poppy has also been used as a natural sedative for thousands of years. In more modern times, inorganic bromides began to be used as synthetic sedatives in the 1850s. Valerian was often mixed with these compounds to enhance their effect (Cazin, 1885). By 1903, the synthetic barbiturates were introduced, and they have since become extremely popular.

One of the most popular sedative drugs ever is diazepam, better known as Valium, which was introduced in 1964. It is used to control anxiety and tension and to relieve muscle spasms. Despite the similarity in names between valerian and Valium, there is no chemical similarity between the two, though valerian's long-standing use as a sedative may have been suggestive to those who first named Valium. Another sedative that has become popular in the last few years is Xanax, a drug from the same class of compounds as Valium and Librium.

While strong, synthetic sedatives such as Valium have definite applications, they also have troublesome side effects, including severe dependence (PDR, Wilson), a "drugged" feeling the morning after, and losses in locomotor coordination (Von Eickstedt, 1969). That's why many doctors in Germany prescribe valerian

---

Valerian has been a popular medicinal herb for thousands of years, though it has not always been used as a sedative.

---

preparations for mild to moderate cases of nervousness, anxiety, or insomnia. In the United States, however, the good news about valerian seems not to have arrived yet; doctors here still resort to Valium and Xanax for these conditions.

THE HISTORY OF VALERIAN

Valerian has been a popular medicinal herb for thousands of years, though it has not always been used as a sedative. The ancient Greeks used it for digestive and urinary tract disorders, and it has been an important herbal remedy in traditional Ayurvedic (from India) and Chinese medicine. In the West, since the 17th century valerian has gained a reputation as a primary cure for nervous conditions such as epilepsy, hysteria, anxiety, and insomnia.

The word *Valeriana*, the botanical name for valerian, is thought to derive from the Latin *valere* (to be in health) or *valeo* (to be strong), referring either to the plant's powerful healing properties or strong odor, respectively. After a heady whiff of the long-dried root, one would be more likely to believe the second explanation, because the odor of old valerian roots has been likened to that of well-seasoned, dirty socks! Another ancient name for valerian, *phu* (or *fu*), is usually interpreted as an exclamation of disgust at the plant's less than felicitous aroma.

Although most people find the smell of old valerian roots to be nothing short of nauseating, surprisingly, the fresh roots and the

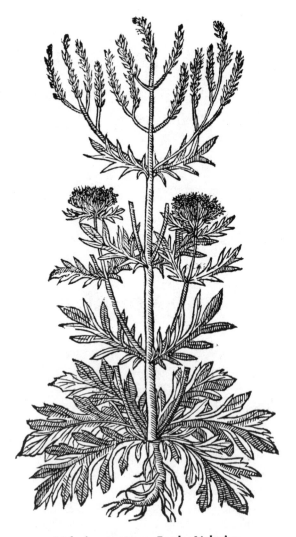

***Valeriana petrea*. Rocky Valerian.**
from *The Theater of Plants*
by J. Parkinson, 1640.

Valerian

essential oil have a sweet, musky odor that is quite pleasant. Fresh valerian was used by some ancient cultures as a perfume (Grieve, 1931). Modern research has shown that some of the sedative activity of valerian may be due to its odor-causing constituents, so I like to add freshly distilled essential oil of valerian to tinctures and powdered extract tablets to enhance their relaxing and sleep-promoting effects.

Valerian was not generally used as a sedative and sleep aid until the late 16th century, when the Italian botanist Fabius Columna (1567-1650) reported that it cured him of epilepsy. By the 18th century, valerian was firmly established as a primary nerve remedy (Woodville, 1790). Since then it has left a long legacy in official drug books, pharmacopoeias, formularies, and dispensatories, continuing into the 20th century. For a complete review of the history of valerian, refer to the appendix.

Valerian has left a long legacy in official drug books, pharmacopoeias, formularies, and dispensatories, continuing into the 20th century.

Valerian was especially popular in the 19th century for nervous conditions in women, called the "vapors," which were characterized by a wide range of symptoms such as chills, waves of heat or cold, involuntary movements, tossing of the body, hiccoughs, anxiety, panic, fears, etc. Valerian was prescribed to women of all ages, from pre-pubescent girls to menopausal women. Indeed, it has even been called "the Valium of the 19th century."

Valerian was listed in most official drug books in both England and the United States until only 40 years ago. As late as 1967, it was still official in the pharmacopoeias of Austria, Belgium, Brazil, Chile, Czechoslovakia, France, Germany, Hungary, Yugoslavia, the Netherlands, Poland, Portugal, Roumania, Russia, Spain, Switzerland, India, and Japan (Todd, 1967).

VALERIAN TODAY

Valerian is currently used widely in Europe, and its popularity is rapidly growing in the United States, Canada, Australia, and New Zealand. In many of these countries, valerian preparations can be purchased in drug stores, and in some places they are even prescribed by medical doctors.

Modern herbalists use valerian and valerian preparations as antispasmodics, sedatives, and sleep aids for a number of conditions, including:

✓ emotional stress
✓ muscle pain
✓ menstrual and intestinal cramps
✓ bronchial spasms
✓ lingering coughs
✓ tension headaches
✓ insomnia
✓ nervousness and restlessness
✓ anxiety
✓ withdrawal from benzodiazepines (Xanax, Valium) (Hölzl and Godau, 1989).

In Europe, valerian is also used as a homeopathic remedy (in dilutions of 3X and 6X) and is recommended for hypochondria, excitability, restlessness, sleeplessness, bloating, and sexual excitement (Boericke, 1927). Note that valerian may cause diuresis (urination) in some people, so it is not always suitable as a sleep aid for those who must urinate frequently during the night (Renner, 1937).

Other uses for valerian include **nervous heart conditions**, **children's anorexia** caused by over-excitement (taken 1/2 hour before meals), "**inner unrest**", **trembling**, and **stomach complaints** (Koch, 1982). A German valerian-hops preparation has been recommended as a good daytime sedative, because it does not reduce reaction time (Bühring, 1976), while another German preparation called *Recvalysatum Burger* can be helpful in cases of hysteria, neurasthenia, excitement, anxiety, and psychosomatic illness induced by stress.

Valerian has also been used for **chronic digestive disturbances**, **stomach cramps**, **colic, diarrhea**, and **bloating** (especially when caused by emotional and physical stresses or coffee, alcohol, and nicotine abuse), as well as for **Grave's** (Parkinson's) **disease**, **excitable conditions during menstruation (PMS)**, and in children for **bed-wetting** and **roundworms** (Madaus, 1938).

So how does valerian help with all of these seemingly different ailments? In scientific terms, we know that valerian's sedative effect works in two ways:

1. By depressing activity in some centers of the central nervous system (brain and spinal cord); and

2. By causing the smooth (involuntary) muscles in the uterus, colon, and bronchial passages to relax.

As you can see, valerian's action on all nervous, stress-related, and psychological conditions is probably a result of its effect on the central nervous system, while its relaxing action on smooth muscles makes it useful in relieving menstrual cramps, digestive and bowel disorders, and possibly mild forms of asthma.

In holistic terms, the body is considered to be an ecosystem of interrelated functional processes. Thus, if an individual has problems falling asleep, which is a symptom of a nervous system imbalance, we would not be surprised to see digestive and hormonal imbalances (such as PMS) as well, since the nervous system is intimately connected with the digestive and endocrine systems. We will take a closer look at herbal energetics, which help

Major Effects of Valerian

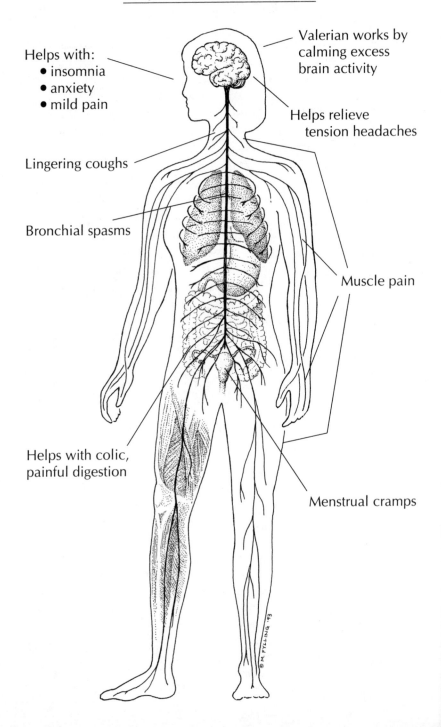

Helps with:
- insomnia
- anxiety
- mild pain

Lingering coughs

Bronchial spasms

Helps with colic,
painful digestion

Valerian works by
calming excess
brain activity

Helps relieve
tension headaches

Muscle pain

Menstrual cramps

© M. FYLLING '93

explain how valerian works in holistic terms, in the next section. Table 1 summarizes the main uses and effects of valerian.

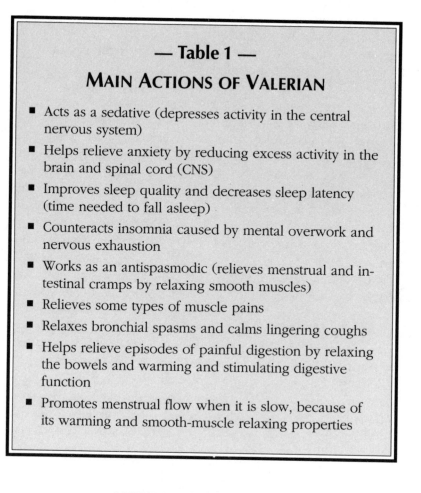

— Table 1 —

MAIN ACTIONS OF VALERIAN

- Acts as a sedative (depresses activity in the central nervous system)
- Helps relieve anxiety by reducing excess activity in the brain and spinal cord (CNS)
- Improves sleep quality and decreases sleep latency (time needed to fall asleep)
- Counteracts insomnia caused by mental overwork and nervous exhaustion
- Works as an antispasmodic (relieves menstrual and intestinal cramps by relaxing smooth muscles)
- Relieves some types of muscle pains
- Relaxes bronchial spasms and calms lingering coughs
- Helps relieve episodes of painful digestion by relaxing the bowels and warming and stimulating digestive function
- Promotes menstrual flow when it is slow, because of its warming and smooth-muscle relaxing properties

HERBAL ENERGETICS

In most systems of traditional healing, such as Traditional Chinese Medicine (TCM) and Ayurveda (from India), herbs are categorized not only by their action on certain diseases, but also according to the qualitative way in which they affect bodily processes. These functional characteristics of herbs are called *energetics*. In TCM, for instance, herbs may be warming or cooling, drying or moistening, stimulating or calming. Significantly, traditional medicine also looks at the energetics of the patient to see whether his or her metabolism and other bodily processes are too slow or too fast, too warm or too cold, too dry or too moist. Once this constitution has been determined, then an appropriate herbal combination can be prescribed. This is in contrast to allopathic medicine, which often considers diseases as independent events that have no individual context.

In energetic terms, valerian is generally considered to be warming, dispersing (removes blood stagnation and hence pain), and slightly drying. Thus it works best for individuals who have internal coldness and/or stagnant energy, because it antidotes these conditions. Even when a person has some internal heat (which manifests as headaches, mouth sores, or dermatitis), valerian may still be beneficial, provided there is also deficiency (weakness, low energy, thin or underweight body). For the latter case, valerian should be combined with herbs such as rehmannia (cooked style) or anemarrhena, both of which strengthen the body and reduce heat.

I have found that nervous problems such as insomnia and anxiety can be due either to a general weakness (deficiency) of the body, or to an excess condition in which there is ample vitality that is out of control. In the first case, which is common among people over 40 and in the elderly, it is necessary to add strengthening herbs and foods to the total program for best results. In the second, which is common among the young (especially teenagers and people in their early 20s), it is important to cool and sedate, and to avoid stimulants of any type (such as coffee or cola drinks). Note that valerian will usually be less effective for people in this second class.

DIET

The importance of diet cannot be overstated. For nervous system and sleep disorders due to *deficiency*, I strongly recommend a diet of mostly cooked foods, especially whole grains, legumes, and vegetables. In extremely deficient conditions, fish or chicken may be added 3 or 4 times a week—and this regimen should be strictly followed for lasting success. For *excess* conditions, on the other hand, a whole-foods diet like the one above can be adopted, but seasonal, raw, organically-grown fruits and vegetables should be added, since these are cooling (fish and chicken are optional). For both conditions, however, I recommend strong moderation with red meat, which is very warming, for both health and environmental considerations.

Valerian and valerian preparations can be useful for nearly any nervous or sleep imbalance, with the addition of appropriate diet and herbs that help make valerian energetically suitable for the individual (see Table 2 next page).

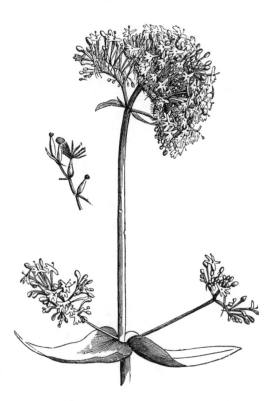

Centranthus ruber
from *School Botany*
by J. Lindley, 1862.

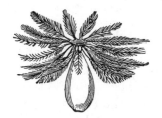

Ripe fruit

— Table 2 —

DIETARY RECOMMENDATIONS FOR NERVOUS CONDITIONS

Condition	Constitutional Condition	Dietary Recommendations
Sleeplessness, nervousness, anxiety, depression	*deficiency*: weak adrenals, easily fatigued, small pulse, tongue with no coating and reddish color, internal coldness accompanied by avoidance of cold weather and cold foods; preference for warm or hot weather, and hot drinks	a warming, building diet: mostly cooked grains (organic white basmati rice, millet, etc.), well-soaked and cooked small beans (aduki, mung), fish, chicken; celery and beet- top tea
Sleeplessness, nervousness, anxiety	*excess*: heat, headaches, full pulse, red tongue with yellow coating, solid energy, accompanied by preference for cool weather and cool drinks	a cooling, cleansing diet: 50% *cooked* grains, legumes, vegetables, and 50% *raw* fruits and vegetables; strictly avoid stimulants (coffee, cola drinks, chocolate), and refined sugar in any form (even honey, fruit juice, and dried fruits) and spicy foods
Hypertension	*excess* condition: dizziness, ringing in the ears, feeling of heat in the upper body	warm celery juice, garlic oil capsules, watermelon; avoid stimulants, red meat, fatty and fried foods; cooling, cleansing diet

FORMULAS FOR COMMON AILMENTS

I have found that valerian blends very well with a number of other relaxing herbs. Herbs often work synergistically, making formulas more effective than single herbs. The skillful formulation of herbal ingredients can also help counteract any unwanted side effects of single herbs. Table 3 provides herbal formulas for common ailments, while Table 4 lists important information about the herbs used in these formulas.

— Table 3 —

VALERIAN FORMULAS FOR COMMON AILMENTS

Condition	Herbs	Dose, Duration of Use
Menstrual cramps	blend with cramp bark, motherwort, chamomile and a little ginger	*tea*: 1 tsp/cup of herb blend, simmer 10 minutes, steep for 20 minutes; drink up to 3 cups/day as needed *tincture*: 1-2 dropperfuls in a little water or tea 2-3x daily *Dry extract* (tablets): 1-2 tablets 2-3x daily as needed
Insomnia or poor sleep	blend with hops, California poppy, hawthorn, and passion flower; for kids add chamomile and/or catnip	same as above; *Note*: take valerian preparations 1/2 hour before bedtime for sleep
Mild anxiety	blend with hops, California poppy, wild oats	same as above
Restlessness (unrest)	add wild lettuce and passion flower	take liquid extract drops throughout the day (20-40 drops/dose) as needed
Bronchial spasms, coughs	combine with thyme, grindelia, yerba santa, mullein, and marshmallow root	liquid extract form is effective for resinous expectorant herbs like yerba santa; 1-2 dropperfuls/dose several times daily; dilute if the taste is too spicy or strong
Painful digestion	combine with a "bitters" formula (i.e., gentian, artichoke, orange peel, cardamon, etc.), or simply with skullcap and wild lettuce (equal parts), and a little ginger to taste	1-3 dropperfuls of the liquid extract taken 15 minutes before meals, or just after eating; bitter tonics work best when taken for up to 2 months or more; they are often taken on an ongoing basis

➡

Tics, muscle spasms, twitches	blend with skullcap, wild oats, and passion flower	must be taken over a period of several months; same dose and schedule as for menstrual cramps, above
Anxiety with weakness, dizziness, feelings of spaciness	combine with astragalus, dong quai, reishi, and a little licorice	decoct (simmer) for 30 minutes, steep for 15, and drink 2-3 cups daily; use the herbs in soups and stews often; tincture and powdered extract as in menstrual cramps section
Nervousness with depression	combine with St. John's wort and lemon balm oil (no more than 3 drops of oil per cup)	use St. John's wort in tincture or standardized tablets or capsules *only*—add liquid extract drops to tea or water

Recommended Dose Schedule

I generally recommend the following dose amount and schedule for valerian preparations:

Average Dose

Tincture: 40-120 drops (1-3 dropperfuls) 3x daily or as needed
Tea: 1 tsp/cup simmered for 15 minutes, steeped for 10 minutes—1-3 cups daily
Powder. (in "00" capsules): 2-3 caps 3x daily as needed
Powdered extract (in tablet form): 1-2 tablets as needed

— Table 4 —

IMPORTANT SEDATIVE AND SLEEP-PROMOTING HERBS

Herb	Major Active Constituents	Pharmacology— Major Actions [temperature, energy]	Main Uses
Valerian *Valeriana officinalis*	iridoid glycosides (valepotriates), essential oil, un-	central nervous system sedative, soporific (induces sleep), im-	tension, anxiety, sleeplessness, insomnia, "inner

	known water-soluble compounds found in the tea	proves quality of sleep [warming and drying; bitter, astringent, and sweet]	unrest, trembling, nervous stomach, hysteria, neurasthenia" (with other tonic herbs)
Hops *Humulus lupulus*	a very complex mixture of volatile oil components (0.3-1%), resinous bitter components (humulone, etc.—3-18%), flavonoids, phenolic acids & tannins (3.5%), estrogenic substances, minerals (8%)	antispasmodic, sleep-inducing and calming, mildly anxiety-relieving [warm; bitter]	helps with sleeplessness due to tension or anxiety, to relieve headaches, tension, mild anxiety
Passion Flower *Passiflora incarnata*	in the whole flowering plant, a series of alkaloids, including harman, harmine, harmaline and harmol; many flavonoid glycosides such as rutin, vitexin, luteolin, orientin, kaempferol, etc.	central nervous system depressant, hypotensive (lowers blood pressure), pain-relieving, sedative [neutral; salty]	can help relax the imagination in people who are worried or anxious, in my experience; helpful for people who have elevated blood-pressure, especially when due to mental tension and worry
Catnip *Nepeta cataria*	essential oil (ca. 0.3%), especially containing ∂- and ß-nepetalactone, plus nerol, thymol, citronellal, carvacrol and others; iridoid glycosides, including epid-eoxyloganica acid; tannins	antispasmodic, sedative, diaphoretic [cool; spicy]	helps increase elimination through sweating, especially during colds and flu, where it can help reduce fever; mild sleep-inducing herb, safe for children; mild digestive tea and antispasmodic for colic, intestinal cramps

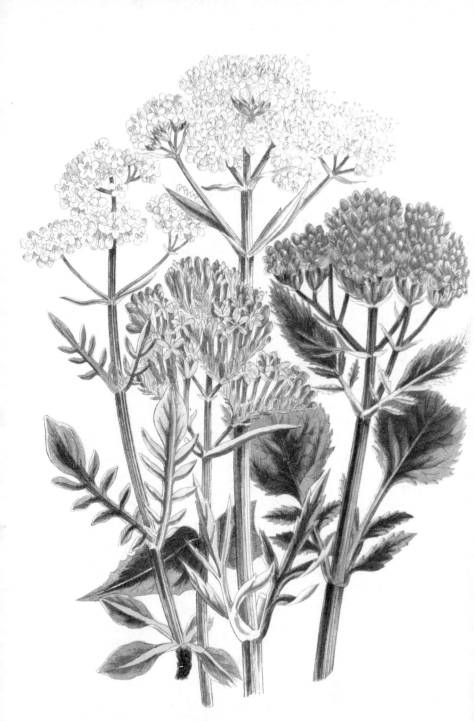

Centranthus ruber   *Valeriana dioica*   *V. officinalis*   *V. pyrenaica*
from *Flowering Plants of Great Britain*
by A. Pratt, ca. 1890.

Skullcap *Scutellaria lateriflora*	flavonoid glycosides such as scutellarin, iridoid glycosides (catalpol), volatile oil, waxes and tannins	antispasmodic, sedative, anticonvulsant [cool; bitter]	as a tincture or powdered extract, it is often used to reduce nervous tension, to relieve hysteria, and to mitigate epileptic or other spasms; also as a mild bitter tonic; must be used long-term; little scientific work has been done on the herb
Wild Lettuce *Lactuca virosa*	the dried milky juice of this plant contains the sesquiterpene lactone, lactucin, and flavonoids, such as quercitin and coumarins	considered a mild sedative and sleep-inducing herb, antispasmodic for coughs; its bitter properties give it mild digestion-stimulating actions [cool; bitter]	in cough syrups, in tincture, or solid-extract form for mild sleeplessness and restlessness; possibly useful in pain-relieving formulas
California Poppy *Eschscholzia californica*	the whole plant contains a number of alkaloids, including eschscholtzine, ionidine, sanguinarine, californidine, and a number of others	Some of the alkaloids have been found to have relaxing effects on the muscles of the uterus; antispasmodic (muscle relaxing), anxiolytic (anxiety-relieving), and pain-relieving [cool; bitter]	the tincture or powdered extract can help relieve pain and produce a calm sleep, helping one to relax; also useful for relieving mild anxiety and spasms in coughs or intestinal cramps; it is considered safe for children
Asafoetida *Ferula assa-foetida* L.	about 40-60% resin (with asaresinotannols + esters), volatile oil (with polysulphides, sulphated terpenes, vanillin, etc.), gum	antispasmodic, carminative, nerve sedative	used in cough preparations, especially for chronic coughs, asthma, colic, and in formulas to help relax hysterical or nervous people ➡

	(ca. 25%), coumarins (umbelliferone, foetidin, etc.)	[hot; spicy]	
Poppy seeds *Papaver somniferum*	small amounts of alkaloids (codeine and morphine) have been detected in humans following ingestion of poppy seeds	mild sedative, hypnotic, anodyne [neutral; oily]	tincture or powdered extract of poppy seeds has a mild sleep-inducing, pain-relieving, and relaxing effect
Lady's Slipper Orchid *Cypripedium bulbosum*, C. sp. *Note: Lady's slipper orchids are listed as "Rare and Endangered" in some states	not well-studied; possibly glycosides, essential oil, resin, and tannin	sedative, nervine, mild hypnotic [warm, slightly bitter]	helps to relieve mild anxiety, headaches, nerve pain and relax one during emotional stress
Lavender *Lavandula officinalis*	volatile oil, coumarins; some triterpenes and flavonoids	antispamodic, sedative, antidepressant [warm; spicy]	used for spasms, nausea, headaches, and emotional exhaustion
Kava *Piper methysticum*	kawain, methysticin, dihydrokawain, dihydromethysticin, and yangonin; contains both lipid- and water-soluble compounds	narcotic, sedative, psychotropic, and nervine [warm; spicy]	helps one feel calm and relaxed; enhances mental activity and communication
Wild Oats *Avena fatua*	proteins, C-glycosyl flavones, avenacosides, fixed oil, starch, etc.	nervine tonic, sedative, anti-addictive [neutral; demulcent]	strengthens the nerves; good for insomnia from nervous exhaustion

| St. John's wort *Hypericum perforatum* | dianthrone derivatives, flavanols, xanthones, coumarins, phenolic carboxylic acids, carotenoids, and essential oil components | tonic nervine, sedative, anti-inflammatory, and antidepressant

[cool; salty] | for nervous imbalances with depression; nerve pain and inflammation |

MODERN STUDIES ON VALERIAN

Valerian's effectiveness as an herbal sedative has been demonstrated by centuries of popular use and informal clinical observations. But what does modern science have to say about valerian? Clinical research today is much more rigorous than it was 50 years ago. Today doctors and scientists like all studies on drugs to be *controlled* and run *double blind*. In a controlled study, one group of subjects is given the medicine under investigation, while a second group receives a placebo (inert substance such as sugar or starch). Neither group knows what they are getting. The placebo gives a more or less "objective" standard for evaluating the effectiveness of the medicine being tested.

A double-blind study goes even further: not even the doctors who are giving the drugs know which patients are getting the drug and which are getting placebo. Everything is kept "secret" until researchers analyze the results at the end of the study. The purpose of double-blind studies is to prevent doctors from communicating their subconscious expectations to patients via body language and other subtle cues.

Only a few controlled, double-blind studies have been conducted on valerian to date; however, those that have been done have all shown valerian to be an effective sedative. For instance, in one double-blind study patients given a preparation of valerian and hops showed significant improvement in subjective feelings of stress-reduction (Moser, 1981). Another test using the same preparation (Seda-Kneipp) demonstrated improvements in subjective and objective sleep parameters for sleep-disturbed patients (Müller-Limmroth, 1977). That means the people in the study both *said* they sleep better and were *observed* to have slept better according to various objective criteria and measurements, such as EEG readings of brain wave patterns.

Other double-blind experiments using pure valerian water extracts (similar to a tea of the roots and rhizomes) have demonstrated subjective and objective improvement in a variety of sleep parameters. These studies indicate that valerian decreases sleep latency (the time needed to fall asleep); increases sleep quality (subjective), especially with elderly poor sleepers; and does not affect normal levels of nocturnal movement. The researchers who conducted these studies concluded that valerian compares favorably with prescription sedatives such as benzodiazepines and barbiturates (Leathwood et al., 1982; Chauffard et al., 1981; Leathwood et al., 1982b; Leathwood & Chauffard, 1985).

A final study reported a dose-dependent reduction in sleep latency of 50% using a valerian water extract (Balderer & Borbély, 1985). "Dose-dependent" means that small doses of valerian produced small decreases in sleep latency, while larger doses produced proportionately greater reductions.

Interestingly, no currently known active compounds were found in the valerian water extracts mentioned above. Thus the active components in these sleep studies *remain completely unknown!*

Excellent results were achieved in 73% of a group of 120 children who were given Valmane, a standardized blend of active constituents from valerian, for psychosomatic and behavioral disorders. The children experienced symptoms such as hyperactivity, fear, restlessness, sleeplessness, constipation, and headaches. The preparation was nontoxic and well-tolerated (Klick, 1975).

A commercial preparation containing valerian and hops (Biral®-neu) reduced central hyperreactivity of the central nervous system in a test with 20 volunteers. Measurements showed that improvements in depression and anxiety (CIPS-inventory) were not only as effective as a drug therapy but worked faster (2 weeks for the valerian preparation compared to 6 weeks for the drug) and had much fewer side effects (Schellengerg et al., 1993).

CHEMISTRY

As you may have gathered from the last comment above, biochemists still have more to learn about valerian. Nevertheless, even though we don't yet know *all* of the active constituents in valerian, we do know many of them. The three major groups of active constituents identified to date include volatile (essential) oils, iridoid esters (valepotriates), and a small amount of alkaloids. Other as yet unidentified, water-soluble components may also play a role in the herb's activity. In any case, it is still unknown whether valerian's activity resides mainly in one compound, a group of compounds, or a synergistic effect.

. . . it is still unknown whether valerian's activity resides mainly in one compound, a group of compounds, or a synergistic effect.

One important conclusion that has come out of the biochemical research on valerian is that valerian species vary widely in the types and quantities of active constituents they contain. In other words, different species have different amounts of essential oils and valepotriates. It has also been found that valerian preparations differ greatly in their effectiveness, depending on the type of preparation, age of the herb, age of the extract, species, variety and chemical race of the plant, and growing conditions of the plants used. For instance, some herbalists who use valerian (including Ayurvedic doctors) have reported that the herb can produce a *stimulating* effect, depending on the patient's condition and constitution, as well as on the age and species of the dried herb. In my experience, the old roots, especially, are more likely to produce such a stimulating effect.

Another important aspect of valerian's chemistry concerns the valepotriates, which have been the subject of intensive research since they were first discovered in 1966. These have aroused some concern, since they have been shown to be cytotoxic (poisonous to cells) and mutagenic (causing mutations) in high concentrations. However, I hasten to add that valepotriates are highly unstable. Since they decompose quickly under the influence of heat and moisture, *most commercial preparations of valerian contain very few of the original valepotriates.* Also, valepotriates are broken down rapidly by the hydrochloric acid in the stomach (Wagner, 1980).

TOXICITY

Although no acute toxicity has been reported for valerian, some people who take large doses (over 1-2 tsp. of tincture per dose) on a constant basis may experience minor side effects such as headaches, lethargy, excitability, uneasiness, insomnia, and/or disturbances in heart activity (List & Horhammer, 1979; Roth et al., 1984; author's experience). In my experience, such side effects are more common with long-dried roots than with fresh or fresh-dried roots and rhizomes.

Regarding the valepotriates mentioned above, their toxic effects are only an issue in highly concentrated extracts (usually powdered) in which valepotriate levels have been boosted beyond their natural levels of about 2%. Furthermore, although valepotriates have been shown to be toxic when given to animals in large amounts (Koch, 1982), they have demonstrated no toxicity in the doses prescribed for humans (Tortarolo et al., 1982). No doubt this is due, in part, to the fact that valepotriates break down rapidly in the digestive tract and are not well absorbed by the intestines.

COMMERCIAL PREPARATIONS

Valerian is one of the most common ingredients in "nervine", sedative, and sleep-promoting herbal formulations (Ross & Anderson, 1986). It is usually blended with hops *(Humulus lupulus)*, passion flower *(Passiflora incarnata)*, and skullcap *(Scutellaria*

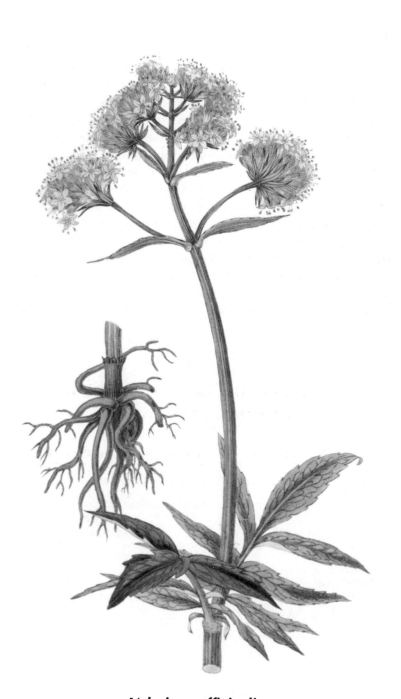

Valeriana officinalis
from *Medical Botany*
by Stephenson & Churchill, 1834.

lateriflora), among others.

Valerian can be purchased singly as a tincture, or in capsules as a simple powder, or in concentrated extract form as capsules or tablets (see Table 5). Tinctures (hydro/alcoholic preparations) have been very popular in Europe, but recently tablets and capsules containing standardized extracts have taken precedence. In the United States, valerian preparations can be found in most natural food stores and herb shops, and occasionally in drug stores.

Seventy-nine commercial German preparations of valerian are mentioned by one author (Koch, 1982). Some modern preparations combine valerian with purified amino acids and other isolated nutrients. One of these products, a mix of valerian and L-tryptophan, was found to be an effective sedative in animal studies (Hara, 1985). In the United States, L-tryptophan has been banned for sale on the natural food market due to an incident involving human illness resulting from an L-tryptophan product which was contaminated with small amounts of a potent toxin.

— Table 5 —
PROS AND CONS OF VARIOUS VALERIAN PREPARATIONS

Preparation	Description	Positive Points	Possible Drawbacks
Tea	rhizome, roots	inexpensive	taste
Tincture	alcoholic extract	moderately priced	activity may vary; contains alcohol, which may be objectionable to some people
Standardized extract	content of essential oil components or valepotriates guaranteed	more consistent quality and effect	usually more expensive

QUALITY CONSIDERATIONS

The quality of the herb that goes into an herbal product is of utmost importance. As the saying goes, "garbage in, garbage out."

To determine the quality of an herbal product, look to see whether the herbs are *certified* organically grown—it should say so on the label. If you are buying bulk herbs and no sign is posted, ask the manager of the store. Organic valerian is readily available, and there are a number of reputable companies that sell products containing it. Buying certified organic products assures you of getting high-quality, uncontaminated herbs. Remember, too, that products made from fresh or fresh-dried valerian are likely to be stronger and smoother-acting than ones made from old valerian.

Today, in countries worldwide, quality control is a vital aspect of an herb industry. Even for personal use, a potential herb user wants to be certain that she or he is taking the correct herb, one which has the expected activity and effects. With the modern techniques of thin-layer chromatography and high-pressure liquid chromatography, among others, it is possible to "look inside" a given herb sample and detect the presence or absence of active or toxic compounds. It is also possible to "fingerprint" a given species of plant to aid in the detection of adulteration. Fortunately, more products are now available that use such quality-control methods.

HOME CULTIVATION

Valerian is easy to propagate, grow, and harvest. It is not particular about soil type and will grow in many climates—hot or cold, wet or dry, and at a variety of altitudes—provided it gets sufficient water and nitrogen. *Valeriana officinalis* can often be purchased from a local nursery. Place several plants into soil that is loose, well-cultivated, and rich. Add compost from kitchen scraps and yard trimmings, or buy commercial organic compost and work it into the bed. The plants will spread and fill a small bed in one or two years, at which point they can be thinned and washed for drying or immediate use. Only the roots and underground stems (called rhizomes) are used for medicine. The young spring and early summer green leaves can be eaten raw in salads or steamed as greens (they are quite tasty).

Time of Harvest

Valepotriate content decreases in autumn, while essential oil content is variable and is not linked to valepotriate levels (Pethes & Verzárné-Petri). According to one report, the best time to harvest the rhizome is at the end of September of the first year, in the morning, during cool weather. At this time, the roots have reached about 85% of their maximum root-weight and contain 0.8% valepotriates and 0.5% essential oil (Wagner et al., 1972). However, other studies have reported the highest amount of root constituents (in Egypt) in the winter (Rashid, 1973); of essential oils in the spring (Rashid, 1973); and of essential oils and alkaloids during the flowering and fruit-bearing phases of summer and early fall (Kornievskii, 1971).

Based on all this, I would say that valerian is best harvested in the fall or early spring.

Drying Methods

When drying any herb, the best method is the one that dries the plant in the shortest time (to prevent enzymatic breakdown of active constituents) without overheating.

One initial study found maximum preservation of active valepotriates when drying without forced air flow at 32-35 deg. C. (90-95 deg. F.), while the best preservation with forced air flow (0.05 m3/min) was seen at 60 deg. C. (140 deg. F.). On the other hand, a second study determined maximum preservation of essential oils occurred at 40 deg. C. (104 deg. F.) with an air flow rate of 0.05 kg/s.m.[2]. Considering both active fractions and the fact that low to moderate levels of valepotriates are desirable, it appears that the best overall method of drying is at 40 deg. C. with an air flow rate of 0.25 kg/s.m.[2] (Lutomski et al.).

Extraction Methods

For home use, valerian rhizomes and roots (preferably fresh-dried) can be extracted in alcohol and water according to the methods given in the *United States Pharmacopeia* (USP), 11th ed. After grinding the herb to a coarse powder, macerate one part (by weight) of the powder in 5 parts (by volume) of the menstruum for two weeks, shaking daily. Then press out and filter for use. The menstruum consists of 1 part distilled water to 3 parts 95% grain alcohol (or 100 proof vodka if grain alcohol is not available). If a stronger preparation is desired, extract the drug up to a concentration of 1:3 (herb powder:menstruum).

When using fresh, *undried* rhizomes and roots, mash the herb and blend it with enough menstruum so that the final product will have 2 inches of clear liquid above the "herb mash." Let the mixture steep for 2 weeks, press, then filter for use.

The most effective extraction method includes pre-moistening the drug in water before final extraction. Shaking or vibrating the drug and menstruum decreases extraction time from 4 days, under normal conditions, to only 30 minutes. To extract the highest possible amount of valeric acid, a major essential oil component, repeat 3 successive extraction processes of 1.6 hours, 1 hour, and 1 hour, respectively (Gromova, 1975).

Stability of Constituents

Even though high levels of valepotriates may be undesirable (as in a purified extract), nonetheless, extremely low levels are also undesirable, because they make for a weaker preparation. Since valepotriates break down rapidly after valerian has been milled and macerated in a hydro-alcoholic menstruum, extraction and storage in *olive oil* may boost stability (Schäte, 1972). Ethyl alcohol is a moderately effective solvent for extracting most of valerian's active constituents (Petricic, 1978), but most valepotriates will still disappear after 1 year (Danielak, 1971).

STRESS-REDUCTION TECHNIQUES

No work on nervous conditions would be complete without a discussion, however brief, of stress-reduction techniques. Regular, moderate-to-intense aerobic activity is key to releasing stress and tension. When the body's "flight or fight" mechanism (sympathetic branch of the autonomic nervous system) is constantly being activated by noise, stress, stimulants, and emotional intensity, the muscles are prepared for action. But if instead of *acting* (exerting ourselves) we sit at a desk all day or watch TV, then this energy can become congealed, leading to stiff, painful muscles; poor circulation; and eventually chronic internal tension and depletion of vital energy.

The following activities help keep a body stress-free and relaxed. If you are not already on a program of relaxation and aerobic activity, why not start with 15-20 minutes of walking and deep breathing today? You will find that you become addicted to feeling good, and you will be much more relaxed in all your other activities, as well. When you start a program for the first time, make sure to work into it slowly, over a period of several weeks, so as not to shock or strain yourself. Please note that people with severe ailments (such as heart conditions) should check with a qualified physician before undertaking any exercise program.

Exercises to Reduce Stress

Walking is one of the best (and certainly the cheapest) health tonics available. Recent research shows that walking can be as effective as running for stress-reduction and providing the health benefits of aerobic exercise.

Running is an excellent antidote to built-up stress and is beneficial for all bodily processes. Endorphins, compounds that relieve pain and can lead to a feeling of euphoria and well-being, are released in the body while running. Note that it is best to avoid running on pavement, which is hard on the knees.

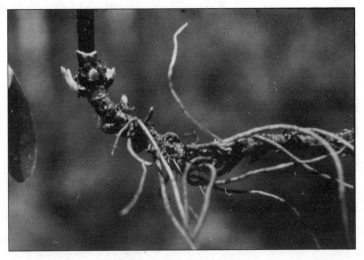

Valeriana sitchensis rhizome

Dancing can be a vigorous aerobic workout that helps release both emotional and physical energy. All of our creative impulses can be activated in this ancient human expression, leading to a total body experience of the highest sort.

Singing is excellent for letting go of unexpressed emotions and helping to dissipate negative feelings such as anger or grief. It also helps oxygenate the blood, tissues, and organs.

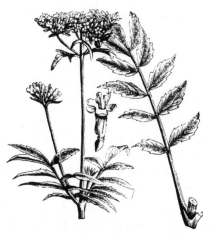

Valeriana officinalis
from The Plant Compendium
ed. Jim Harter, 1988.

Biking can distract the mind with ever-changing scenery and provide good mental release as well as aerobic exercise.

Yoga exercises can be immensely beneficial for stress-reduction. To enhance their value, add daily meditation and breathing exercises.

Deep Breathing is excellent for calming the mind and body, and it can help strengthen the nervous system. Practice breathing into the "hara," the space below the navel, for 10-20 minutes once or twice a day.

Meditation consists of focusing the mind on the breath, repeated sound or words, or uplifting image. This induces deep relaxation, improves concentration, frees the mind from turmoil, and insulates one from stress and over-excitement. Meditation is a most highly recommended "non-activity" for anyone of any age or state of health!

Tai Chi is an ancient Chinese form of active physical meditation, through which one's mind and body are harmonized. It is a gentle form of exercise which can nevertheless bring great strength and balance.

See the Resources section for books and programs that use these activities (and non-activities!) in total healing programs.

BOTANY

Taxonomy

Valerian is a member of the family Valerianaceae Batsch., of the genus *Valeriana* L., which comprises 200 species worldwide (Bailey, 1976; Hickey). The genus is distinguished from others in the family by having 3 stamens; a small, nectar-bearing sac at the base of the corolla; an epigynous, feathery pappus; and a one-chambered ovary. Other closely related genera include *Valerianella* Miller (corn salad), *Centranthus* DC (Jupiter's beard), and *Nardostachys* DC (nard), all of which are commonly grown for medicine or as ornamental subjects (Rendle, 1963).

Although many species of *Valeriana* have been used for medicine, the wild species is considered to be stronger than the garden varieties (Greene, 1824). The most common species for medicinal purposes is *Valeriana officinalis* L. Unless otherwise noted, in the rest of this appendix valerian will be taken to refer to *Valeriana officinalis* L.

Description

Valerian is described as a perennial garden herb that grows to 5 feet high from a short rhizome, and is sometimes stoloniferous, producing new plants from horizontal runners. The grooved stalk is usually simple or slightly branched above. The opposite leaves are smaller above and are all divided into 7-10 entire or dentate-serrate pairs of leaflets. The small, fragrant, pinkish or whitish (sometimes lavender or red) flowers have sympetalous, irregular tubular corollas, often spurred at the base, and 3 stamen. The inflorescence is a terminal compound cyme (or corymb). The inferior ovary is crowned with a feathery pappus.

Range and Habitat

Valerian species are indigenous to most parts of Europe and parts of northern Asia, ranging from Spain to Iceland, to the North Cape and Crimea, to the coast of Manchuria in northern Asia (Flückiger & Hanbury, 1879; Tutin et al., 1964). Family members are rare in Africa and North America, but do occur in South America (Pratt, ca. 1890). The plant is cultivated in many parts of the world, spreading rapidly by means of runners, and can escape.

Synonyms

Synonyms for valerian include *Valeriana sylvestris* (Pharm. Lond., Edinb., Dod.), *Valeriana sylvestris* major (C. Bauh. Fin. p. 164, Tourn.), *Phu germanicum* (Fuchs.), *Phu parvum* (Matth.), *Valeriana foliis pinnatis, pinnis dentatis* (Hal. Hist. Stirp. Helv. n., 210), *Valeriana officinalis* (Lin. Gen. Plant., p. 44, Hudson. Flor. Ang., p. 12).

Etymology of Nomenclature

The name valerian, or *Valeriana*, first appeared in the literature between the 9th and 10th centuries, though its origin is uncertain. Pliny and Dioscorides, ancient Greek authors, called *V. tuberosa* "valeriane" (Pickering, 1879), however, the word *Valeriana* is thought to derive from the Latin *valere* (to be in health) or *valeo* (to be strong), referring either to the plant's powerful healing properties or strong odor, respectively. Some claim it was named after Valerius, who may have first used it in medicine (Paxton, 1849; Jaeger, 1972).

Two other names are known for valerianaceous plants, *nard* and *phu* (or *fu*). The first may be derived from the Sanskrit *nalada*, meaning "odorant", giving rise to the Hebrew *nerd* (Levey, 1966). Phu or fu is usually interpreted as an exclamation of disgust with the strong smell of long-dried valerian root. As early as 1515, *Valeriana* was repeatedly said to be synonymous with phu, a plant described by Sibthorp and now accepted as *V. dioscorides* (Flückiger & Hanbury, 1879; Gunther, 1933; Pickering, 1879; Thompson, 1830).

Many names for valerian have been used in Europe through the centuries. Common English names for the plant are theriacaria, amantilla, herba benedicta, and setwell. The last was used by the common people but was said to more properly be applied to zedory (Gerard, 1633). The German name is *baldrian*, the French, *valeriane*. Most north and central European names derive from "Vandal's Root", the meaning of which is unknown, but probably referring to its use by the 4th century invading Teutonic tribe known as Vandals.

HISTORY OF USE

Hippocrates (460-370 B.C.) used a kind of valerian as medicine (Fuchs, 1895-1908). Theophrastus of Eresos, a student of Aristotle (370-286 B.C.), mentions *V. dioscorides'* use as perfume (Theophrastus).

In general, the ancient Greeks used the valerian species primarily for their bitter and aromatic qualities, not for their sedative effects. Dioscorides, originator of the modern Materia Medica (54-68 A.D.), mentions several members of the valerian family, which he recommends for digestive problems, flatulence, nausea, stagnant liver, and urinary tract disorders. Dioscorides categorizes the nards as being warming and drying, and as tasting bitter, astringent, and sweet. The Greeks also used valerian species as an emmenagogue, antiperspirant, and antidote to poisons, as well as for vaginal yeast infections and for potions and warming ointments (Gunther, 1933).

Pliny's (23-79 A.D.) *Natural History* mentions 12 varieties of nard, among them Gallic nard, *Valeriana italica*, and phu. His uses closely follow those of Dioscorides. Galen, the last influential Greek physician and pharmacist (131-201 A.D.), in a rare reference prescribes valerian to induce sleep (Pickering, 1879).

Nardostachys jatamansi, a member of the valerian family, is the ancient spikenard mentioned in the Bible. It was used as a perfume for flavoring foods and for healing oils and unguents, especially for the head (Ainslie, 1826; Sanyal, 1984).

After the early Greek authors, only a couple of major contributions were made to medicine during the ensuing millenia, notably the Arabian school (8th-13th centuries) and the school of Salerno (1050-1220). In his Formulary (9th century), Al-Kindi of Baghdad calls nard sunbul and recommends it "to cure pustules in the mouth, protect the soft gum from heat, to cure insanity, and to strengthen the breathing." He used Indian nard in a stomachic formula, "wild" nard in the *nosh-daru* electuary to "make one happy," and Celtic nard (*V. celtica*) in an enema to warm the bladder and kidneys (Levey, 1966).

Starting in the late 15th century and continuing through the 17th century, herbalism flourished throughout Europe. The great herbals of the time recommended valerian for a variety of conditions (see Table 6).

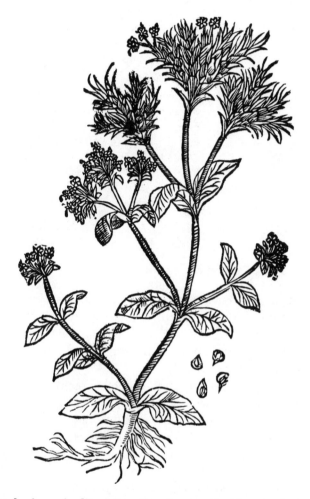

Valeriana indica sive Mexicana. **(Indian Valerian)**
from *The Theater of Plants*
by J. Parkinson, 1640.

— Table 6 —

VALERIAN IN THE GREAT HERBALS

Herbal	Date	Uses
Matthiolus	1544	Diuretic, anodyne, emmenagogic, carminative; for coughs, asthma, and internal injuries
Dodoens	1554	A gargle for throat inflammations
Turner	1568	To perfume clothes
Gerard	1597	Root extraction as diuretic, for jaundice, cramps, convulsions, bruises; leaves good for ulcers and mouth and gum sores
Parkinson	1640	Boil with licorice, raisins, and aniseed for short-windedness, coughs, to keep away the plague, and expel wind from the belly; boil in white wine, place drop in the eye to "take away dimness of sight." Decoction for colds, especially after over-heating the body
Culpeper	1649	"Under the influence of Mercury." Otherwise, quotes earlier writers

Valerian was also used widely as a pot herb and seasoning for meats and stews (Gerard). Surprisingly, back then it was deemed to have a sweet and agreeable flavor, inspiring the poet Chaucer to sing: "But he himselfe was swete as any roote of licoris, or any Setewall" (Pratt, 1890).

An unusual use valerian found during this period was as bait for rattraps, since rats and cats are said to be attracted by the plant's smell. In fact, it has even been suggested that the Pied Piper of Hamelin used valerian roots to woo rats (Grieve, 1931).

The modern application of valerian for the nervous system was not "discovered" (or re-discovered) until the late 16th century. As the story goes, the Italian botanist Fabius Columna (1567-1650), finding no successful treatment for his epilepsy, finally followed Dioscorides' prescription of valerian and was cured. Woodville (1790) also recounts this story, but adds that Columna later suffered a relapse.

By the 18th century, valerian was firmly established as a primary nerve remedy (Woodville, 1790). Since then the plant has been so popular that it is impractical to cite all the literature on it. Valerian has left a long legacy in official drug books, pharmacopoeias, formularies, dispensatories, and materia medicas, continuing into the 20th century (see Table 7). It was especially popular in the 19th century for nervous afflictions in women, called "the vapors," which were described as including anything from "noises in the head, chills, waves of heat or cold, eccentric impatience, thrills which compel involuntary movements, tossing of the body and hiccoughs" to "anxiety, panic, fears, etc." (Trousseau and Pidoux, 1880). Valerian was prescribed to women of all ages for such conditions, from pre-pubescent girls to menopausal women.

— Table 7 —

VALERIAN IN OFFICIAL AND UNOFFICIAL COMPENDIA

UNOFFICIAL WORKS

Year	Work	Preparations	Indications
1733	*New English Dispensatory*	ingredient in Venice treacle; powder	Nervous cases, hysteria; *V. sylvestris* (wild var.) stronger than *V. hortensis* (garden var.)**
1747	*Pharmacopoeia Universalis*	powder in wine, tincture	Sudorific, diuretic, poor sight, asthma, cough, liver stagnancy, jaundice, coldness. Tincture for nervous conditions, epilepsy
1790	Edinburgh New Dispensatory	powder, infusion, tincture; dose = a scruple to a dram	Nervous system debility, epilepsy. To induce sleep, especially during fevers (irregular results)
1802	Cullen's Materia Medica	powder, tincture	Use in large doses as anti-spasmodic, for hysteria
1814	A Family Herbal	tea, oil, wine, tinc., electuary (1 oz powder in orange peel syrup; take in rosewater)	Many refs. for epilepsy; jaundice; failure of action due to poor quality; disease of thorax, stomach, uterus; tetanus; "sordid ulcers"

1821	Thatcher's New American Dispensatory	powder, infusion	Dose=scruple to dram; 2-3 X/day, increase as the stomach can bear. Wild var. on Ohio river as good as *V. officinalis*.
1830	Coxe's American Dispensatory	powder	Essential oil most active; decoction is not active
1833	*London Dispensatory*	extract, infusion, tincture	Hypochondriasis, use with mace or cinnamon to moderate taste
1880	Trousseau's Materia Medica	powder	The "vapors" in women
1898	King's American Dispensatory	fluid extract, infusion	This major Eclectic work recommends valerian as a "stimulant-tonic", for cases of "enfeebled" cerebral circulation." However, modern research shows valerian slows the brain's metabolism.
1931	Grieve's Modern Herbal	several	Nervous overstrain, after-effects of narcotics, nervousness during air-raids; for poor eyesight, insomnia, cardiac palpitations, cholera; and as soap and perfume

OFFICIAL WORKS

Year	Work	Preparations	Indications & Notes
1618	*London Pharmacopeia*	infusion, tincture, ammoniated tincture	None given (Indian and Celtic Nard also listed); valerian official from 1618-1948
1820	*U.S. Pharmacopeia*	tincture, ammoniated tincture	Official from 1820-1936
1830	*U.S. Pharmacopeia*	tincture, ammoniated tincture	Antispasmodic, tonic, emmenagogue; dose 1-4 gm
1888	*National Formulary*	fluid extract, ammoniated tinc.	Official from 1888-1946

Valerian

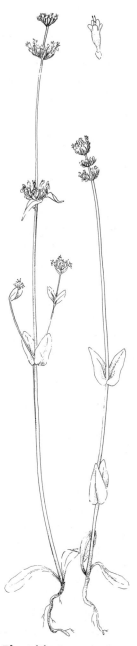

Plectritis ssp. congesta

**NOTE: In most English works written between the late 16th and early 19th centuries, *V. sylvestris* was reported to be a wild kind of valerian growing in England that has stronger medicinal properties than the garden variety, *V. hortensis.* Linnaeus combined these two varieties into one species, *V. officinalis.*

Valerian was listed in most official drug books in both England and the United States until only 40 years ago. In 1967, it was still official in the pharmacopoeias of Austria, Belgium, Brazil, Chile, Czechoslovakia, France, Germany, Hungary, Yugoslavia, the Netherlands, Poland, Portugal, Roumania, Russia, Spain, and Switzerland. *V. wallichii* DC. was official in India, *V. officinalis* var. *latifolia* in Japan (Todd, 1967). Various valerian preparations are currently used in Europe as antispasmodics.

In Ayurveda, the ancient system of healing from India, *Jata mamsi,* a species of valerian, is used to cure poisoning and internal burning sensations (Dash, 1987). Today *V. jatamamsi* (=*V. wallichii*) is used interchangeably with valerian in the Indian herb trade. It is considered tonic, stimulant, antispasmodic, diuretic, deobstruent, emmenagogic, stomachic, and laxative. Scientific experiments have demonstrated antiarrhythmic, anticonvulsant, and hypotensive effects, as well as measurably depressant action on the central nervous system (CSIR).

In Traditional Chinese Medicine (TCM), *V. jatamamsi* has been known for centuries as "one of the five odorous plants." The plant is considered deodorant, carminative, stimulant, and useful for headache, skin problems, mental depression, ascarids, and malaria (Perry, 1980; Shih-Chen, 1578).

CHEMISTRY

Through the early 20th century, the sedative effect of valerian was usually ascribed to the essential oil (especially the ∂-methylpyrrylketone), until later tests showed the essential oil accounts for only 1/3 of the plant's total activity (List & Hörhammer, 1979). Today the important active compounds of Valerianaceae plants are divided into 3 groups:

1. the volatile oil, which contains active sesquiterpenes;
2. non-glycosidic iridoid esters exhibiting many different variations on a basic structural theme; and
3. a small amount of alkaloids.

Two conditions especially call for more study of these compounds. First, valerian preparations differ greatly in their effectiveness, depending on the type of preparation, age of the herb, age of the extract, species, variety and chemical race of plant, and growing conditions of the plants used. North American species have hardly been studied, and in general valerian species vary widely in their chemical race, varieties, and constituents (Hazelhoff et al., 1979; Hendriks & Bruins, 1980). For instance, valerenic acid, a proven active sesquiterpene, could not be detected in *V. wallichii, V. edulis, V. mexicana,* or *Centranthus ruber* (Chadha, 1976; Rashid, 1973).

Second, one major group of active compounds, the valepotriates, are known to be cytotoxic and mutagenic. By using species that are lower in these possibly toxic compounds, or by adjusting extraction methods, it may be possible to minimize their negative impact, if any.

The majority of characterization performed over the last 60 years on the constituents of *V. officinalis*, its varieties, chemovars, and several other species, along with a brief summary of their major activity, is presented in Table 8. The percentage of a given compound or fraction is assumed to be of the dry roots of *V. officinalis*, "European variety", unless otherwise noted. References for pharmacological activity are included.

Perhaps the most noticeable aspect of valerian roots is their strong aroma. This is more remarkable for the fact that the fresh root has little smell, except when scratched or crushed. It is known that as valerian dries, an enzymatic change occurs during which isovaleric acid (the odorous compound) is released from one of the several compounds with which it is esterified—either the valepotriates or from bornyl valerate (Kraemer, 1915).

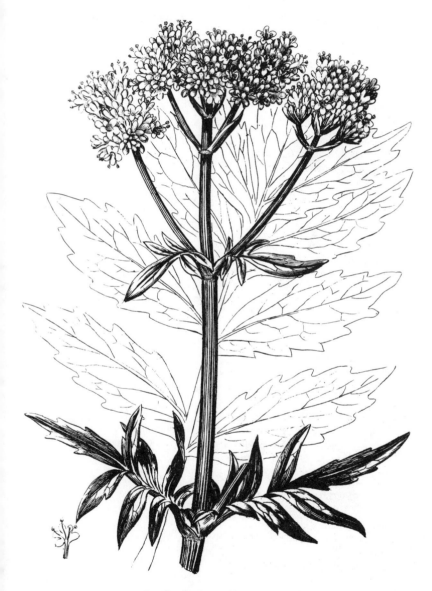

Valeriana officinalis
from *Medical Botany*
by W. Woodville, 1790.

Valerian

— Table 8 —

THE MAJOR CONSTITUENTS AND PHARMACOLOGICAL ACTIVITY OF VALERIAN

Constituent & References	Activity and References
Carboxylic acids	
(Houghton, Morvai & Molnar-Perl, Wagner, 1972, Rücker, 1979) 21 free and esterified carboxylic acids, including mainly isovaleric, malic, acetic, stearic, and palmitic acids.	—
Essential Oil Components Percent composition varies widely with species, variety, and growing conditions (Kionka, Stoll et al., 1957); most likely plays a role in activity (Hendriks et al., 1981).	
V. officinalis (European) Contains usually less than 1% v/w (Rücker, 1979; Violon et al., 1984) Russia: 0.4-1%; plants at higher elevation gave higher % (Savin)	Reduction of spontaneous activity in animals (Stoll et al., 1957); tincture fortified with essential oil counteracted breakdown of valepotriates (Wagner, 1980).
*Monoterpenes	
12 compounds (Stoll et al., 1957), mainly bornyl acetate (31%), isovalerate; also caryophyllene, ∂- and ß-pinene, camphene, l-borneol, l-myrtenol, limonene, myrcene, phellandrene, (Gunther & Althausen; Koch, 1982), carvacrol, carvone (8.2%), thymol (4.3%) (Corsi), terpinene, terpinolene, p-cymene, a-fenchene.	The various physiological effects of monoterpenes reviewed by Wagner & Wolf
Terpene esters: bornyl formate, 1-mertenyl acetate, 1-myrtenyl-isovalerianate Terpene alcohols: l-borneol, valenol, l-myrtenol Terpene ketones: valeranone, valerenone, kanokonole	—

Valmane ® (80% didrovaltrate, 15% valtrate, 5% acevaltrate) From *V. wallichii*	Tranquilizing effect in mice at 31 mg/kg, improvement in coordination. Less aggressiveness, anxiety, and restlessness in cats (von Eickstedt & Rahman; von Eickstedt); spasmolytic activity (Wagner & Jurcic).
Vpt$_2$ (50% valtratum, 25% valeridin, hypnotic (Petkov & Manolov).	Myorelaxant, anticonvulsive, 3% valechlorin)
Valepotriate fraction	Spasmolytic (Schätte, 1971); acts on amygdaloid body (Hölm); inhibits complement, may be useful for autoimmune disease (van Meer); sedative, increases GABA (Dunayev); sedative, anti-arrhythmic (Petkov & Manelov)
1. Valepotriates (with a closed epoxy ring)	
Monoene type (one double-bond) Didrovaltrate	Breakdown product, valtroxal more sedative (Veith et al.); spasmolytic (Wagner & Jurcic; Hazelhoff et al., 1982); inhibits efferent impulses to hippocampus (Hölm).
isovaleroxyhydroxydidrovaltrate	—
Diene type (two double-bonds)	Sedative effect at 100 mg/kg, but lower than its breakdown product, homobaldrinal (Wagner, 1980); sedative at 0.5 mg/kg (Hölzl & Fink); spasmolytic (Wagner & Jurcic, Hazelhoff et al., 1982); changes EEG pattern (Fink).
isovaltrate (0.25-0.75% total in root) (Violon et al, 1983)	Lower activity than homobaldrinal (Wagner, 1980); spasmolytic (Hazelhoff et al., 1982)
acevaltrate	—
2. Valepotriate-hydrines (open epoxy ring)	
Monoene type Valechlorine (didrovaltrate-hydrin)(Popov).	—

Diene type
Valtrate-hydrin B1
Valtrate hydrine B2
Acetoxyvaltrate hydrine   Sedative at 4 mg/kg
(Hölzl & Fink).

3. Valepotriate-glycosides

Monoene type
Valerisodatum, patrinoside, kanokoside B,
kanokoside A

4. Breakdown products

Baldrinal
homobaldrinal   Greater activity than valtrate
                                    & isovaltrate (Wagner, 1980)

Valtroxal   Sedative (Hölzl & Fink);
                                    slight sedative activity
                                    (Veith et al.)

---

*Sesquiterpenes
Valerenic acid   Spasmolytic (Stoll, 1957); 50
                                    mg/kg, sedative in mice;
                                    valerenic acid characteristic for
                                    V. officinalis (Hendriks, 1981;
                                    Hendriks, 1985); CNS activity
                                    decreased by inhibition of
                                    GABA breakdown (Riedel et al.)

Valerenal   50 mg/kg sedative in
3-16% (Hendriks & Bruins)   mice (Popov et al.)

Valeranone   Hypotensive, tranquilizing in
0-18% sometimes undetectable   mice (Arora & Arora); sleep
(Hendriks & Bruins);   prolonged, tranquilizing in rats
much higher in N. jatamansi   (Popov et al.); 100 mg/kg dose
(Hörster et al.)   prevented ulcers, had sedative
                                    activity (Hendriks et al, 1981);
                                    antispasmodic by musculo-
                                    tropic effect (Hazelhoff
                                    et al., 1982) anticonvulsive,
                                    hypotensive, and sedative;
                                    affects serotonin and
                                    noradrenaline levels (Hendriks
                                    et al., 1985)

Valerenol, hydroxy valerenic acid, —
valerenyl esters (several) (Bos et al.)

Pacifigorgiol (0.7-8.6% of essential oil) (Bos et al.)	—
Guaiol, eudesmol, valerenone, elemol 2-12% (Hendriks & Bruins), acetoxy-valerenic acid, hydroxyvalerenic acid, bisabolol, cadinene, caryophyllene, curcumene, ergnophylene, kessane, ∂-valene, ß-valene, y-valene, δ-valene, azulene (Stoll et al.; Rücker, 1979; Hänsel & Schultz, 1982); maali alcohol(Stoll et al.), patchouli alcohol, ß-ionone (Rücker & Tautges); Faurinone (Bos et al.); ∂-Kessyl alcohol 9-10% (Hendriks, 1980)	—

*Triterpenoids

ß-sitosterol

Alkaloids

Chatinine and valerianine at 0.01% were first discovered by Walliczewski (1891) (Franck)	
Actinidine and isovaleramide (Buckova; Johnson & Waller)	Antibiotic
∂-methylpyrrylketone (Cionga) dipyridylmethylketone (Janot et al.)	Anaesthetic, sedating (Cionga)

Miscellaneous Constituents

isoeugenyl-isovalerate (Hendriks, 1981)	Minor activity (Hendriks, 1981)
Hesperetinic, behenic acids (Stoll & Seebeck)	—
Chlorogenic acid, caffeic acid (Fichter)	—
Luteolin, quercetin derivatives, (diosmetin, etc.), kaempferol (upper parts) (Rybal'chenko et al.)	—
Palmitic, oleic, stearic, linoleic, linoleic, linolenic and arachidonic acids (Bullock)	—
Choline (Szentpetery)	—
The amino acids GABA, tyrosine, and glutamine (Hänsel & Schultz)	—
The enzymes catalase, oxidase, peroxidase, lypase	—

➡

Sugars, starch, tannin, resins, and rubber (Rücker)	—
The seeds of *Valeriana* species contain a wide variety of fatty acids— *V. officinalis*: 60% linoleic acid + 15-21 others (Dolya)	Good food and energy source in areas of large populations

Other Species

V. officinalis var. *latifolia*
  (=*V. angustifolia*)
Contains 0.5-6.0% v/w (Hikino); compounds were detected, e.g., acetate (51%), camphene (16%), ∂-pinene (7%), ß-pinene (6.5%), carveyl acetate (5.5%), limonine (2%), dihydrocarveyl acetate (2%) (Long et al.); the valepotriates, kanokosides A, B, C, D (Endo & Taguchi); kessane derivatives (Hikino et al.)

For a review of pharmacological activity of the monoterpenes, see Wagner & Wolf (1977); essential oil has protective effects against pulmonary edema in rats, also prevented arrhythmia, contraction of coronary vessels (Cun-kuan)

kessoglycol diacetate

Prolongs sleeping time in rats, decreases motility (Takamura, et al., 1973; Takamura et al., 1975; Hikino et al.)

V. celtica L.
44 compounds identified, mainly isovaleric acid, seychellene, patchouli alcohol (53.4% total) (Bicchi)

V. edulis sp. *procera* Meyer
(*Valerian "mexicana,"* commercial)
Root contains valtrate, didrovaltrate, isovaltrate (Roumeliotis & Unger; Hazelhoff et al. 1982)

Antispasmodic effect (Hazelhoff et al. 1982)

V. wallichii D.C.
Thies first isolated iridoids from this species. The flavonoid linarinisovalerianate (Thies; Chari et al.). A review on the constituents of the essential oil, acids, and others (Rashid et al.). Also see (Chadha).

Crude alkaloid fraction

Antibacterial, gram + (Rashid, et al.)

Nardostachys jatamansi
Contains 4% v/w essential oil (Rücker et al.)

Patrinia scabiosaefolia Fisch
0.1% volatile oil, primarily composed of patrinene, isopatrinene; also isopentanoic acid, saponins, (patrinosides—considered the major active fraction) (Chang & But)

Liquid extract, dry extract and volatile oil, but not the non-volatile fraction, showed sedative and hypnotic activity in animals and humans; 406 patients showed 50% improvement in insomnia; no acute toxicity was observed at 1500 times normal (Hochun et al.) (For a review see Mannenstaetter et al.).

---

*Monoterpenes
∂-pinene (14.5%), maaliol (12%), borneol acetate (7.2%), bomeol (4.5%), p-cymene (1.2%), etc. (Wang & Niu)

---

*Sesquiterpenes
Jatamansone (valeranone) (Govindachari et al.; Krepinsky et al.)

(see *V. officinalis*)

Centranthus ruber
High in valepotriates (5-7%) (Mannenstaetter et al.; Adzet et al.; Marekov) The leaves show up to 1% valepotriates —none in *V. officinalis* leaves (Hölzl & Jurcic) Contains only very small amounts of essential oil.

Decreased motility in mice (Adzet et al.)

Review of new constituents:
gentioside, gentioflavoside, gentioflavine (an alkaloid), gentiopicroside, swertiamarin, gentianine, gentianidine, 8 new valepotriates (Marekov).

North American species:
V. sitchensis sp. *scouleri* (Pacific valerian) (plants collected from the wild at locations around northern California and Oregon). Valepotriate content of dry root (1.12%), leaf (0.033%). Various *Plectritis* spp. have less than 0.08% in roots (Förster et al.).

Note: Although the valepotriate levels in *V. sitchensis* are similar to *V. officinalis*, there is a larger concentration of essential oil in one population of *V. sitchensis* that was tested by the author using TLC (unpublished results). Due to the recent emphasis on the essential oil as an active fraction, the Pacific valerian may be a promising one for future commercial cultivation.

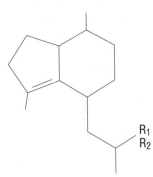

1. Valerenal, valerenic acid

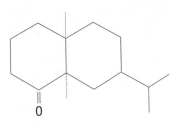

2. Valeranone

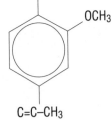

3. Isoeugenyl-isovalerate

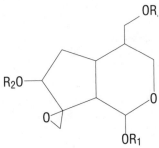

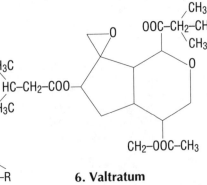

4. Valtrate

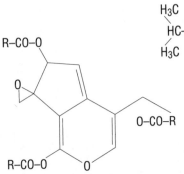

5. Valepotriate

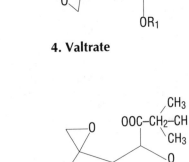

6. Valtratum

VALEPOTRIATES

Because the essential oil was shown to account for only approximately 1/3 of the total activity of valerian, the search continued for active constituents. In 1966, the first valepotriates were discovered—bicyclic iridoid esters isolated from *V. wallichii* and *Centranthus ruber* (Thies, H. 1966). The name *valepotriate* was derived from "valerian-epoxytriester." Later work enumerated many new valepotriates (Thies, 1968; Thies, 1967; Thies et al., 1981; Thies et al., 1974), leading to patents and synthetic derivatives (Thies, 1971; Thies, 1970). Information on the biosynthesis of iridoids with an epoxide structure is available (Voigt et al., 1978).

Generally, valepotriates have shown spasmolytic, sedative, and anticonvulsant activity (Thies, 1970; Finner et al., 1984; Marekov et al., 1983). It has been suggested that valepotriates interact with the essential oil constituents of a similar base skeleton to produce nervous system activity (Hazelhoff et al., 1979). Since their discovery, many European valerian products have been standardized to them.

There are several structural variations among the valepotriates, according to the acid substituents esterified to the -OH groups on the main iridoid skeleton (or lack thereof) (Thies, 1981); presence of an epoxide group; number and position of double bonds in the main nucleus; and presence or absence of glycosidic sugars (Houghton, 1988). Three main iridoid types are found in the *Valerianaceae*, one as breakdown products upon exposure to heat, moisture, or acid. The first two types contain a closed epoxy ring and are very unstable. Most of these compounds are non-glycosidic, unlike most other iridoids in the plant kingdom, and have been isolated from only Valeriana and Centranthus.

As with the essential oil, the amounts and types of valepotriates vary widely among *Valeriana* species (Trzhetsinskii et al., 1984): 0.2-1%, rarely 1.5-2%, in *V. officinalis* (Marekov et al 1987); 5-7% in *Centranthus ruber*; 7-8% in some South American species (Marekov et al., 1983). Mostly valepotriates are concentrated in the rhizome and roots, although at least one species *(V. kilimandascharica)* has a high percentage in the leaves (Dossaji, & Becker, 1981).

PHARMACOLOGY

Early research on valerian focused on the essential oil's depressant effect on the central nervous system of frogs and rabbits (Binz, 1876), as well as on cats, dogs, birds, and mice (for review, see Madaus or Koch). However, although these early studies contain a wealth of circumstantial evidence, they do not meet the more rigorous standards of modern research, because the individual compounds were not known, and the quality and identity of the herb samples were not reported or controlled (Houghton, 1988). Nonetheless, well-designed recent studies on humans have corroborated valerian's depressant effect on the CNS (Krieglstein and Grusla, 1988).

On the other hand, some herbalists who use valerian claim that the herb can also produce stimulating effects, depending on the age and species of the dried herb, as well as on the patient's constitution and condition. This stimulating effect was noticed by the Eclectics, and in Ayurvedic medicine it is used as such. This points again to the possible need for standardization and to keep in mind the species' differing chemical constituents when determining pharmacological activity (Table 8, Chemistry section).

The search for the active components of valerian reached a kind of plateau with the discovery of the valepotriates, which lately have been accepted as the plant's major active components. However, this is by no means a foregone conclusion, for several reasons:

1. The **valepotriates** are highly unstable and, under the influence of heat, moisture, or acid (such as the hydrochloric acid in the stomach), decompose quickly into baldrinal and homobaldrinal. Thus, *most commercial preparations of valerian contain very few of the original valepotriates.* However, baldrianal, homobaldrianal, and other breakdown products show activity in some tests (Wagner, 1980)—indeed, sometimes even stronger activity than their parent compounds (Veith et al., 1986).

2. **Water extracts** of valerian, containing no valepotriates (which are not water-soluble) and little essential oil, still have shown sedative effects and have improved sleep in humans. A possible interaction between an active valerian fraction and the GABA-benzodiazepine-barbiturate-receptor complex has been postulated (Koch, 1982; Hänsel et al., 1981).

3. The **essential oil** of Japanese *V. officinalis* var. *latifolia* shows higher sedative activity than Chinese and Nepalese variants with high amounts of valepotriates. This may be due in part to the strong sedative effect of the kessane derivatives, which comprise a major portion of the essential oil (Hikino et al., 1980). The main active compounds in European valerian are currently thought to be valeranone, valerenic acid, and valerenal (Houghton, 1988).

4. Recent studies (1988) equating central-nervous system sedation *only* with the efficacy of valerian suggest that the valepotriates and the major essential oil constituents shown to be active in the past have no effect on the CNS. These researchers did find that *Valeriana* contains central depressant compounds; however, they were not identical with those discussed in the past. Specifically, they tested the whole plant extract, valtrate, didrovaltrate, homobaldrinal, valerenic acid, valeranone, and the volatile oil. All fractions were separated from a dichloromethane extract, so some of the original water-soluble compounds may have been discarded before activity testing (Krieglstein & Grusla, 1988).

Thus, for the moment, it appears that valerian's sedative effect is caused by a combination of depression of some centers of the CNS and direct relaxation of smooth muscle (Houghton, 1988). The most likely active compounds are essential oil components, the valepotriates (iridoid esters), and unidentified water-soluble components.

The few well-controlled clinical trials that have been conducted on valerian are summarized in the section entitled "Modern Studies on Valerian", in the beginning of this book.

CLINICAL APPLICATIONS

Clearly, valerian's major application is as a sedative, especially as a potential substitute for stronger synthetic sedatives, such as Valium and Xanax, which can have undesirable side effects. As discussed in the beginning of this book, many German doctors already prescribe valerian preparations for mild to moderate cases where doctors in this country still resort to Valium and Xanax (Weil, 1989). However, herbalists in the United States currently use valerian extensively for its sedative and antispasmodic action against emotional stress, muscle pain, menstrual and intestinal cramps, lingering coughs, bronchial spasms, tension headaches, insomnia, nervousness, and restlessness (Moore, 1979; Anderson, 1989; author's experience). One clinical herbalist especially recommends it *ad lib* to break dependency on pharmaceutical antidepressants (Anderson, 1989). A recent study showed that the sesquiterpene alcohol, ketone and valepotriate fractions of valerian extracts can displace benzodiazepines (the class of compounds to which Xanax and Valium belong) from their receptor binding sites in animal brain cells (Hölzl and Godau, 1989).

Several authors have noted that valerian products produce diuresis before taking full effect, so they are not always suitable for people who urinate frequently during the night (Renner, 1937). Valerian is warming in energetic terms and can have a stimulating effect on people with heated conditions or hot constitutions. Tierra (1988) says it is best suited for patients with cold, nervous conditions.

Fresh or fresh-dried roots are generally considered superior to long-dried roots (Moore, 1979; Anderson, 1989; author's experience). Dosages vary: 30 drops to 1/2 tsp. of fresh root tincture (Moore, 1979); up to 1/3 - 1/2 tsp. frequently (every 1/2 hour) of fresh wildcrafted plant for severe pain, or up to 1 tsp. for insomnia (Anderson, 1989); or, in this author's experience, up to 1 tsp. of 1:3 tincture, especially in combination with other sedative herbs. One German herbalist has recommended up to 3 tsp. of the tincture per dose (Weiss, 1988); however, in the author's experience this may cause headaches and stomach upset in some patients. It is likely that Weiss used tinctures made from long-dried rhizomes, which are often considerably weaker than fresh or fresh-dried roots or rhizomes.

TOXICITY

Although valerian has had a long history of use, it is not known for certain whether prolonged use of the herb could result in chronic or cumulative toxicity. No acute toxicity has been reported, though with constant use there can be minor side effects such as headaches, excitability, uneasiness, insomnia, and disturbances in heart activity (List & Horhammer, 1979; Roth et al., 1984).

Very large doses may cause central paralysis, lessening of heart-beat, and decrease in intestinal motility and tone, for which the recommended first aid is gastric lavage, charcoal powder, and sodium sulfate (Glauber's salts) (Roth et al., 1984).

Discussion of valerian's toxicity should focus mainly on highly-concentrated extracts (usually powdered), especially when valepotriate levels are boosted beyond their natural levels of about 2% (in *V. officinalis*). The valepotriates' acute toxicity is low—an LD_{50} of over 4600 mg/kg in mice (orally) for valtrate (Koch, 1982)—but they have shown alkylating, cytotoxic, and mutagenic activity. Since cytotoxicity is sometimes due to the alkylating epoxide ring of some of the major valepotriates, such as valtrate and didrovaltrate (Braun, 1982), valepotriates that do not contain the epoxide group, such as the valepotriate-hydrins and valechlorine (among others), may be of more interest in the future (Koch & Hölzl, 1985). However, these latter types of valepotriates also show less activity—for instance, 8 times less than valtrate in one experiment (Hölzl & Fink, 1984).

Valtrate and didro-valtrate both have shown a high degree of cytotoxicity, however, the C5-C6 double bond is the most important structural feature conferring cytotoxicity, not the epoxide ring (Bounthanh et al., 1983). Other studies have also

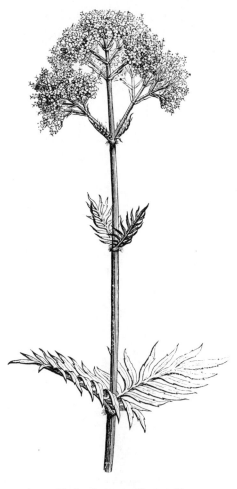

Valeriana officinalis
from *Natural History of Plants*
by H. Baillon, 1871.

demonstrated *in vitro* cytotoxicity (Tortarolo et al., 1982) and mutagenicity (Hude von der, 1985). Because of their reported cytotoxicity, valepotriates have been studied as anti-tumor agents (Bounthanh et al., 1981). However, tests for this effect rendered poor results (Berger et al., 1986).

Despite the *in vitro* toxicity (on cultured cells) of valepotriates, *in vivo* toxicity has not been demonstrated, even with doses as high as 1350 mg/kg (Tortarolo et al., 1982). Poor absorption and distribution of the compounds is invoked as a possible explanation (Houghton, 1988), but a reduced toxicity due to interaction with other constituents in the whole plant extract cannot be ruled out. Also, it is well known that valepotriates break down quickly and probably do not occur in many commercial preparations, and, likewise, that they are metabolized rapidly in the body (starting with gastric H+, then in the liver) (Wagner, 1980).

Interestingly, the baldrianals (breakdown products) are better absorbed and are also sedating. They have been found *in vitro* to be much less cytotoxic (by a factor of 10) than their parent valepotriates, although *in vivo* their cytotoxicity is much more noticeable than the valepotriates', because they are more readily absorbed in the intestine. Baldrianals have been detected in commercial preparations standardized to valepotriates in levels up to 0.988 mg/dose, which *may pose some cytotoxic concern* (Braun

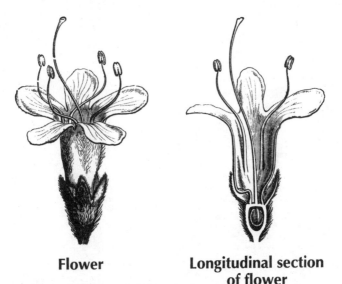

Flower   **Longitudinal section of flower**
from *Natural History of Plants*
by H. Baillon, 1871.

Valerian

et al., 1986).

In the future, commercial valerians that are low or moderate in valepotriates and high in essential oil (as is the case in some varieties of *V. officinalis,* or *V. sitchensis*), may become more popular.

REGULATORY STATUS AND FOOD USE

One species of valerian, *V. officinalis,* has been approved as safe (GRAS) for food use in the United States. Extracts and essential oil of the root are used as flavor components in many major food products, including alcoholic (liqueur, beer) and non-alcoholic (root beer) beverages, frozen dairy desserts, candy, baked goods, gelatins and puddings, and meat and meat products. The highest average maximum use levels are about 0.01% of the extract (no type given) reported in alcoholic beverages and baked goods, and about 0.002% reported for the oil in baked goods (Leung, 1980).

IDENTIFICATION AND ADULTERATION

Valerian, unlike many other herbs, is easy to identify. Its smell is unmistakable and becomes stronger with age. Nonetheless, note that other herbs will adopt valerian's odor when packed with it. Youngken (1950) describes commercial valerian as follows:

"Rhizome vertical, from 2 to 4 cm. in length and from 1 to 2.5 cm. in diameter, entire or usually cut into 2 to 4 longitudinal pieces; externally weak brown to moderate yellowish-brown or dark brown, upper portion with stem bases and leaf scars and frequently with a short horizontal stolon, the outer surface showing numerous slender, brittle rootlets and occasional root scars; fracture of rhizome short and horny; internally brown to moderate yellowish-brown, with a thick bark and narrow central cylinder; odor characteristically valeric acid like, becoming stronger on aging; taste sweetish, camphoraceous and somewhat bitter" [and when the essential oil is high, spicy.]

This author has observed that rhizomes from wild American sources are usually smaller, more sinewy, and less odorous, though they may taste biting.

Since valerian is easy to cultivate and grows abundantly in the wild in many countries, adulteration also poses few problems. The main adulterants of *V. officinalis* are other species of valerian, such as *V. toluccana* and *V. edulis* var. *procera* Meyer from Mexico; *V. phu* L. from the Caucasus; *V. officinalis* var. *latifolia* Miq. and *V. officinalis* var. *angustifolia* Miq. (=*V. angustifolia* Tausch) from Japan; and *V. wallichii* DC (Indian valerian) from the Himalayas. While all of the commercial valerians have their own merits and activity, the active constituents vary widely between species. High valepotriate species, such as Mexican valerian, may be undesirable because of possible toxicity.

. . .rhizomes from wild American sources are usually smaller, more sinewy, and less odorous, though they may taste biting.

Excellent information for the identification of valerian species is available for microscopic analysis (Youngken, 1950; Wallis, 1955; and Jackson & Snowdon, 1968), TLC (Wagner, 1984; Hazelhoff et al., 1979; Rücker et al., 1982; and Vérzarné-Petri, 1977), and HPLC (van Meer & Labadie, 1981; Dossaji and Becker; Tittel, 1978; Freytag, 1983; Wichtl, 1978; Hazelhoff et al., 1979; and Nissen, 1988). For a treatment of the pharmacognosy of Indian valerian (*V. wallichii*), see Mary or Iyengar (still available).

*Note: Contact the Lloyd Library, Cincinnati, Ohio, for help in finding articles from European pharmaceutical journals.

CULTIVATION

Valerian can be easily propagated, grown, and harvested. It is not particular about soil type and will grow in many climates—hot or cold, wet or dry; and at a variety of altitudes (even up to 2400 m)—provided it gets sufficient water and nitrogen.

Valerian is cultivated throughout eastern Europe, in India, America, Japan, and Mexico—but most intensely in England, Belgium, Holland, Russia, and Germany (Youngken, 1950). With overharvesting in the wild increasing, as in India, cultivation will become more important (Mathur, 1988).

Propagation

Propagation is usually accomplished by means of vegetative, generative, or reproductive methods. In parts of Germany, wild plants exclusively are used as starting material.

Since both vegetative and reproductive propagation (the latter common in large commercial operations) stimulate the production of extra blossom-buds, thus reducing the weight of the roots, seeding directly into the field is a better method (Czabajska, 1976).

Germination usually occurs in 5 weeks, at a rate of 80 to 83%, and can be improved by light but not stratification (Dagite, 1969). Seeds lose their viability after 2 years.

The seeds need constant water. Optimum soil moisture content for total yield is between 45 and 60%, however, the essential oil content is highest between 30 and 45% moisture. Hoeing and spacing 40 x 40 cm between plants will also increase yields and has no effect on essential oil content (Berbec, 1968).

In vitro propagation of *V. wallichii* shoot tips and axillary buds has been accomplished, providing a rapid means of cloning high-constituent yielding plant chemovars (Mathur, 1988). See also Wienschierz (1978) for various methods of cultivating *V. wallichii*.

Several diseases have been reported in *V. officinalis* root cuttings, among them *Verticillium* wilt and *Thielaviopsis* root rot (Gerlach, 1973).

— Table 9 —

OPTIMUM PLANTING CONDITIONS FOR VALERIAN

■ Mid-August sowing without thinning provides the biggest crop (135 q/ha fresh matter). Next best is August planting with thinning (120 q/ha), followed by autumn sowing without thinning (119 q/ha). Sowing at other times of the year produces much less.

■ For dry-land farming, time of planting should be gauged on moisture, which is of critical importance. Where moisture is greater in the fall, plant then.

■ Thinning or widening the distance between plants decreases the yield per acre when the seeds are sown at a density of 3 kg/ha.

■ The content of valepotriates and essential oil is affected only slightly by these different parameters, summer sowing without thinning giving a slightly higher yield of essential oil (from Czabajska, 1976).

Fertilization

Adding nitrogen is important for successful cultivation of valerian (Koch). Fertilizers containing nitrogen, phosphorous, and potassium can significantly increase root weight (Jen, 1973; Jen, 1975) and total yield (Binek, 1980), while one study shows that a nitrogen-potassium fertilizer increases valtrate content by 10% over no-fertilizer conditions (Binek, 1980). Another research group determined the optimum ratio between these nutrients to be $N:P_2O_5:K_2O$, 1:0.75:1 (Golcz, 1975).

The desirability of other nutrient applications depends on soil conditions. For instance, in neutral silty soil, addition of calcium ($CaCO_3$) does not improve yields but does slightly increase essential oil content, whereas in slightly acid sandy soil, $CaCO_3$ substantially improves yields (and again slightly increases essential oil content) (Berbec, 1965). This seems to indicate that valerian favors a neutral pH, which is supported by the finding that adding lime to the soil (to achieve a 0.5 h.a. content) increases root yields by 8% and reduces rhizome yields (Gindic & Seberstov, 1968).

Neither essential oil content nor valepotriate levels appear to be influenced much by varying soil conditions, although valepotriate levels do vary depending on the nutrient supply (Jenö, 1975).

Harvesting

Some researchers feel that the best time of harvest is November to February (Koch, 1982). For commercial harvesting, mechanized harvesting methods have been reported (Eisenhuth, 1966). Drying is accomplished on walls, floors, or by kiln. Larger roots are cut to reduce drying time. (See Quality Control section in the first half of the book for more.)

Tissue Culture

Just as cultured bacteria can be genetically altered to produce useful chemical compounds, like insulin, so plant cell cultures can be grown to produce secondary compounds. A number of medicinal plants have been cultured this way, including *Silybum marianum* (for silymarine) and *Digitalis* (for cardio-active glycosides) (Becker, 1979).

Because of the interest in valepotriates, suspension or callus-cultures of Valerianaceae species have been tried in an attempt to produce these compounds. In one study, *V. wallichii* showed a good yield of valepotriates, while *V. officinalis* did not (Becker, 1979). A further study reported that levels of valepotriates from various *Valeriana* species were 0.5-1.8 g/100g dry weight, and up to 3% in *C. ruber* (Violon, 1984). Other information on this process is available (Milkova, 1989; Mathur, 1987; Förster, 1984).

Valerian plants

Forest Farm
990 Tetherow Rd.
Williams, OR 97544
(503) 846-7269

Taylor's Herb Garden
1535 Lone Oak Road
Vista, CA 92083
(619) 727-3485

Richter's
357 Highway #47, R.R. #1
Goodwood, ONT.   LOC 1AO
CANADA
(416) 640-6677

Valerian Seeds

Abundant Life Seed Foundation
P.O. Box 772
Port Townsend, WA 98368
(206) 385-5660

Richter's
357 Highway #47, R.R. #1,
Goodwood, ONT.   LOC 1AO
CANADA
(416) 640-6677

To order dried valerian

Pacific Botanicals
4350 Fish Hatchery Road
Grants Pass, OR 97527
(503) 479-7777

Blessed Herbs
Rt. 5, Box 1042
Ava, MO 65608
(417) 683-5721

Recommended Books for Healthy Living

Christopher Hobbs   *Foundations of Health*
Deepak Chopra   *Quantum Healing*
Svevo Brooks   *The Art of Good Living*
Bernie Siegel   *Peace, Love, and Healing*
Herman Kauz   *Tai Chi Handbook*
Dr. Yang Jwing-Ming   *The Root of Chinese Chi Kung*
B.K.S. Iyengar   *Light on Yoga*

Recommended Herbal Periodicals

Herbal Gram
P.O. Box 201660
Austin, TX 78720

AHA Quarterly Newsletter
P.O. Box 1673
Nevada City, CA 95959

REFERENCES

Adzet, Par. et al. 1976. Activity of the tincture of *Centranthus ruber*, given orally. *Planta Med.* 29: 305-309.

Ainslie, W. 1826. *Materia Medica (of the Hindoos)*, 2 vols. Reprinted by Neeraj Publishing House, Delhi (1984).

Alleyne, J. 1733. *A New English Dispensatory.* London: for Tho. Astley at the Rose, and S. Austen at the Angel and Bible.

Anderson, Cascade. 1989. Personal Communication.

Arber, A. 1938. *Herbals, Their Origin and Evolution.* Reissued 1986. Cambridge: Cambridge University Press.

Arora, R.B. & C.K. Arora. 1963. Hypotensive and tranquillising activity of jatamansone (valeranone) a sesquiterpene from Nardostachys jatamansi DC. In: K.K. Chen & B. Mukerji (Eds.), *Pharmacology of Oriental Plants.* Pergamon, Oxford, pp. 51-60.

Bailey, L.H. & E.Z. Bailey. 1976. *Hortus Third.* Revised by the Staff of the L.H. Bailey Hortorium, Cornell. New York: Macmillan Publishing Co.

Becker, H. & R. Schrall. 1983. Callus- and suspension cultures of different *Valerianaceae* species, their ability to accumulate valepotriates. *Planta Med.* 36: 228-9.

Benecke, R. et al. 1986. Analysis of plant drugs for residues of organochlorine compounds. Part 2: Identification of residues of DDT and its analogs by gas chromatography on packed and capillary columns and by combined gas chromatography-mass spectrometry. *Pharmazie* 41: 499-501.

Benecke, R. et al. 1986. Investigation of residues of organochlorine compounds in vegetable drugs. Part 2: Confirmation of identity of DDT-type residues by gas chromatography on packed and capillary column and by GC-MS.

Berbec, S. 1965. The effect of different rates of calcium on the growth, yield and quality of raw material of medicinal valerian. *Ann. Univ. M. Curie-Sklodowska, Sect. E.* 20: 233-49.

Berbec, S. 1965. The effect of soil moisture on the growth, yield and quality of the raw material of medicinal valerian. *Ann. Univ. M. Curie-Sklodowska, Sect. E,* 20: 215-31.

Berbec, S. 1968. The effect of spacing and hoeing on the quantity and quality of harvested valerian. *Ann. Univ. M. Curie-Sklodowska, Sect. E,* 23: 323-38.

Berger, M.R. et al. 1986. Study on the tumor inhibitory activity of the valepotriates on transplanted and chemically-induced tumors in the rat. *Arzneim.-Forsch.* 36: 1656-59.

Bicchi, C. et al. 1948. Studies on the essential oil of *Valeriana celtica* L. *J. High Resolut. Chromatogr. Chromatogr. Commun.* 7:213-15.

Binek, E. 1980. The influence of fertilization on the root yield of *Centranthus ruber* DC and the valtrate content.

Binz, C. 1876. About the activity of essential oils. *Arch. Exp. Pathol. u. Pharmakol.* 109.

Birnbaum, G.I. et al. 1978. Stereochemistry of valerenane sesquiterpenoids. Crystal structure of valerenolic acid. *J. Org. Chem.* 43: 272-76.

Boericke, W. 1927. *Materia Medica*, 9th ed. Philadelphia: Boericke & Runyon.

Bos, R. et al. 1983. A structure of faurinone, a sesquiterpene ketone isolated from *Valeriana officinalis*. *Phytochem.* 22: 1505-6.

Bos, R. et al. 1986. Isolation and identification of valerenane sesquiterpenoids from *Valeriana officinalis*. *Phytochem.* 25: 133-5.

Bos, R. et al. 1986. Variations in the essential oil content and composition in individual plants obtained after breeding experiments with a *Valeriana officinalis* strain. *Prog. Essent. Oil Res., Proc. Int. Symp. Essent. Oils,* 16th Meeting Date 1985, 123-30. Edited by: Brunke, E.-J. Berlin: de Gruyter.

Bounthanh, C. et al. 1981. Valepotriates, a new class of cytotoxic and antitumor agents. *Planta Med.* 41: 21-8.

Braun, R. et al. 1982. Valepotriates with an epoxide structure—oxygenating alylating agents. *Deutsch. Apothek.-Zeit.* 122: 1109-13.

Braun, R. et al. 1986. Studies on the Effects of Baldrinalon Hemopoietic Cells in *vivo* , on the Metabolic Activity of the Liver *in vivo,* and on the Content in Proprietary Drugs. *Planta Med.* 52: 446-9.

Buckova, A., 1977. Active principles in *Valeriana officinalis L. Cesk. Farm.* 26: 308-9. (CA 88: 86063z).

Bühring, M. 1976. The effect of valerian-hops preparation on the reaction time of clinic patients. *Der Kassenarzt* 16.

Bullock, K. 1924. Die prüfung von Baldrianwurzel und gewissen anderen aromatischen Drogen. *Pharmaceutical Journal* 113: 109-13. Cambridge: Cambridge University Press.

Cazin, H. 1885. *Traite Pratique et Raisonne des Plantes Medicinales.* Paris.

Chadha, Y.R., Chief Ed., vol. X. 1976. *The Wealth of India.* New Delhi: Publications & Information Directorate, CSIR.

Chang, H.-M. & P. P.-H. But. 1987. *Pharmacology and Applications of Chinese Materia Medica,* 2 vols. Philadelphia: World Scientific.

Chari, V.M. et al. 1977. A 13-NMR Study of the structure of an acyllinarin from *Valeriana wallichii. Phytochem.* 16-1110-2.

Chauffard, F. et al. 1982. Detection of mild sedative effects: valerian and sleep in man. *Experientia* 37: 622.

Cionga, E. 1936. Gegenwart von Pyrryl-a-methylketone in stabilisierter *Valeriana officinalis. C.R. hebd. Seances Acad. Sci.* 200; through CA 29 3770.

Corsi, G. et al. 1984. Biological and phytochemical aspects of *Valeriana officinalis*. *Biochem. System. & Ecol.* 12: 57-62.

Coxe, J.R. 1830. *The American Dispensatory*. Philadelphia: Carey & Lea. (America's first Dispensatory, 1st ed. 1906).

CSIR. 1950-1976. *The Wealth of India*. New Delhi: Publications & Information Directorate, CSIR.

Culbreth, D.M.R. 1906. *A Manual of Materia Medica and Pharmacology*. Philadelphia: Lea Brothers.

Culpeper, N. 1847. *The Complete Herbal and English Physician Enlarged*. London: Thomas Kelly.

Culpeper, N. 1983. *Culpeper's Color Herbal*. D. Potterton, ed. New York: Sterling Publishing Co.

Cun-kuan, X. et al. 1988. Effects of the volatile oil from *Valeriana officinalis* var. *latifolia* on acute experimental pulmonary edema. *Chinese Traditional and Herbal Drugs* 19: 403-6 , 431.

Czabajska, W. et al. 1976. New methods in the cultivation of *Valeriana officinalis*. *Planta Med.* 30: 9-13.

Dagite, S. J. & A.V. Morkunas. 1969. Some biological characteristics of *Valeriana officinalis*. *Trudy Akad. Nauk lit. SSR* 2 (46): B, 69-75.

Danielak, R. 1971. Content of valepotrates in Polish commercial *Valeriana officinalis* raw material and some of its preparations. *Farm. Pol.* 27: 849-52.

Dash, V.B. 1987. *Illustrated Materia Medica of Indo-Tibetan Medicine*. Delhi: Classics India Publication.

Dolya, V.S. 1948. The effect of irrigation on the contents and chemical composition of fatty oils in seeds of some cultivated species of *Valeriana* L. *Rastit. Resur.* 22: 348-51. (CA 105:168939).

Dossaji, S.F. & H. Becker. 1981. HPLC Separation and quantitative determination of valepotriates from *Valeriana kilimandascharica*. *Planta Med.* 43: 179-82.

Dunayev, V.V. et al. 1987. Biological activity of the sum of valepotriates isolated from *V. alliariifolia* Adams. *Farmakol Toxicol* 50: 37.

Eisenhuth, F. 1966. *Valeriana officinalis* breeding and field cultivation with special reference to mechanization. *Herba Hung.* 5: 138-40.

Elbanowska, A. et al. 1975. Investigations of the process of valerian rhizome drying in a screen chamber drying oven. Part II. Analytical evaluation of the crude drug and determination of optimum parameters of drying. *Herba Polonica* 21: 316.

Endo, T. & H. Taguchi. 1977. The constituents of valerian root. The structures of four new iridoid glycosides, kanokosides A, B, C, and D from the root of "Hokkaikisso." *Chem. Pharm. Bull.* 25: 2140-2.

Fichter, M. 1939. Isolierung von Chlorogensäure aus Baldrian. *Pharmac. Acta Helvetae* 14: 163-170.

Valerian

Fink, C. et al. 1984. Activity of valtrate on the EEG of the isolated perfused rat brain. *Arzneim.-Forsch.* 34: 170-4.

Finner, E. et al. 1984. Über die Wirkstoffe des Baldrians. *Planta Medica* 50: 4-6.

Flückiger, F.A. and D. Hanbury. 1879. *Pharmacographia. A History of the Principal Drugs of Vegetable Origin.* London: Macmillan & Co.

Förster, W. et al. 1984. HPLC analysis of valepotriates in the North American genera *Plectritis* and *Valeriana. Planta Med.* 50: 7-9.

Franck, B. et al. 1970. Pyridine alkaloids. 6. Valerianine, a tertiary monoterpene alkaloid from valerian. *Angew. Chem., Int. Ed. Engl.* 9: 891.

Freytag, W.E. 1984 HPLC analysis of valepotriates in the North American genera *Plectritis* and *Valeriana. Planta Med.* 50:7-9.

Fuchs, R. 1895-1908. *Sämtliche Werke* (Collected Works). Munich. Vol. 1, pp. 423, 473; vol. 2, p. 474.

General Convention for the Formation of the American Pharmacopeia. 1930. *The Pharmacopeia of the United States of America.* New York: S. Converse.

Gerard, J. 1633. *The Herbal.* Revised and enlarged by T. Johnson, reprinted by Dover Publications, NY. 1975.

Gerlach, W. & W. Franz. 1973. *Verticillium* Wilt and *Thielaviopsis* Root Rot—two previously unknown diseases of Valerian *(Valeriana officinalis L.). Phytopath. Z.* 76: 172-8.

Gindic, N.N. & V.V. Seberstov. The response of chamomile and valerian to liming. *Trudy vses. nauc.-issled. Inst lekarstv. Rast.* 13: 155-60.

Golcz, L 1975. Nutritional requirements of *Valeriana officinalis* L. *Herba polonica* 21: 171-2.

Govindachari, T.R. et al. 1958. Struktur von Jatamanson. *Chemische Berichte* 91: 908-910.

Greene, T. 1824. *The Universal Herbal.* London: Caxton Press.

Grieve, M. 1931. *A Modern Herbal.* Reprinted by Penguin Books, Middlesex, England.

Gromova, N.A. et al. 1975. Extraction of plant raw material in an extractor press. *Pharm. Chem. J.* 8: 709-71.

Gunther, E. & D. Althausen. 1949. *The Essential Oils,* 4 vols. New York: D. Van Nostrand Co.

Gunther, R.T. 1933. *The Greek Herbal of Dioscorides.* Hafner Publishing Co. 1968.

Hänsel, R. & J. Schulz. 1981. GABA and other amino acids in valerian root. *Arch. Pharm.* 314: 380-1. (CA 94: 188665).

Hänsel, R. & J. Schulz. 1982. Quality control of valerian preparations. 2. Valerenic acid and valerenal as characteristic components of *Valeriana officinalis.* Determination by HPLC. *Deutsche Apotheker*

Zeitung 122: 215-219.

Hara, K. 1985. Hypnotic compositions. *Japanese Patent J.* P. 60,202,825 14 Oct. 1985 4 pp. (CA 104: 56440b).

Hazelhoff, B. et al. 1979. Isolation and analytical aspects of *Valeriana* compounds. *Pharm. Weekbl.*, Sci. Ed. 1: 956-64.

Hazelhoff et al. 1982. Antispasmodic effects of valerian compounds: an in-vivo and in-vitro study on the guinea-pig ileum. *Archives Internat. de Pharmacodyn.* 257: 274-87.

Hendriks et al. 1981. Pharmacological screening of valerenal and some other components of the essential oil of *Valeriana officinalis*. *Planta Med.* 42: 62-8.

Hendriks et al. 1985. Central nervous system depressant activity of valerenic acid in the mouse. *Planta Med.* 49: 28-31.

Hendriks, H. & A.P. Bruins. 1980. Study of three types of essential oil of *Valeriana officinalis* L. s.1 by combined gas chromatography-negative ion chemical ionization mass spectrometry. *J. of Chromatog.* 190: 321-30.

Hickey, M. & C.J. King. 1981. *100 Families of Flowering Plants.* New York: Cambridge University Press.

Hikino, H. et al. 1963. Constituents of Kesso root. *Yakugaku Zasshi* 83: 219-230.

Hikino, H. et al. 1971. Constituents of some cultivated Japanese valerian roots. *Yakugaku Zasshi* 91: 650-6.

Hikino, H. et al. 1980. Study on the efficacy of oriental drugs 18: Sedative properties of *Valeriana* roots. *Shoyakugaku Zasshi* 34: 19-24.

Hochun, L. et al. 1986. Clinical observation and pharmacological investigation of the sedative and hypnotic effects of the Chinese drug rhizome and root of *Patrinia Scabiosaefolia* Fisch. *J. Trad. Chin. Med..* 6: 89-94.

Hölm, E. 1984. Activity of valtratum/isovaltratum and didrovaltratum on the cerebral cortex and subcortical brain areas. Electrophysiological experiments on cats. *Osterreichische Apotheker-Zeitung* 38: 45-6.

Hölzl, J. & K. Jurcic. 1975. Valepotriates in the leaves of *Valeriana jatamansii*. *Planta Med.* 27: 133-9.

Hölzl, J. & C. Fink. 1984. Experiments on the effects of valepotrates on the spontaneous motility of mice. *Arzneim.-Forsch.* 24: 44-7.

Hölzl, J. & P. Godau. 1989. Receptor Bindings Studies with *Valeriana officinalis* on the Benzodiazepine Receptor. *Planta Med.* Abstracts of Short Lectures and Poster Presentations, September, 1989.

Hörster, H. et al. 1977. Valeranone Content in the Different Parts of *Nardostachys jatamansi* and *Valeriana officinalis*. *Phytochem.* 16:1070-1.

Houghton, P. 1988. The biological activity of valerian and related plants. *J. of Ethnopharm.* 22: 121-42.

Iyengar, M.A. 1987. *Study of Crude Drugs*, 3rd ed. Manipal: College of Pharmaceutical Sciences, Kasturba Medical college.

Jackson, B.P. & D.W. Snowdon. 1968. *Powdered Vegetable Drugs*. London: J. & A. Churchill, Ltd.

Jaeger, E.C. 1972. *A Source-Book of Biological Names and Terms*, 3rd ed. Springfield, Illinois: Charles C. Thomas.

James, R. 1747. *Pharmacopoeia Universalis: or a New Universal English Dispensatory*. London: for John Hodges, at the Looking-Glass.

Janot, M.-M. et al. 1979. Contribution to the study of valerian alkaloids *(Valeriana officinalis, L.)* : Actinidine and naphtyridylmethylketone, a new alkaloid. *Ann. Pharmac. Franc* 37: 413-20.

Jeno, B. et al. 1974. Effect of state of nutrient supply and soil type on the common valerian *(Valeriana officinalis* L. ssp. collina Wallr.). II. Changes in volatile oil and valepotriate content. *Herba Hung.* 14: 37-46.

Johnson, R.D. & G.R. Waller. 1971. Isolation of actinidine from *Valeriana officinalis. Phytochem.* 10: 3335-6.

Jones, W.H.S. 1956. *Pliny Natural History*. Cambridge: Harvard University Press.

Kionka, E. 1904. Die Wirkung des Baldrians. *Arch. intern, de Pharmakodyn. et de Therapie* 13:215.

Klich, R. & B. Gludbach. 1975. Verhaltenstorungen im Kindesarter und deren therapie. *Med. Welt.* 26:1251-4.

Koch, H. 1982. *Valeriana officinalis* (Baldrian) Bonn: Bundesfachnerbnad der Arzneimittel-Hersteler e. V. (BHI).

Köch, U. & J. Hölzl. 1985. The compounds of *Valeriana alliarifolia*: Valepotrathydrines. *Planta Med.* pp. 172-3.

Kornievskii, Y.I. & K.E. Koreshchuk. 1971. Seasonal dynamics of the accumulation of the main groups of chemical compounds in *Valeriana stolonifera. Farm. Zh.* (Kiev) 26: 67-70. (CA 75: 31300a).

Kraemer, H. 1915. *Scientific and Applied Pharmacognosy*. Philadelphia: published by the author.

Krepinsky, J. et al. 1962. Structure of the sesquiterpene ketone valeranone. *Coll. of Czech. Chem. Comm.* 27: 2638-53.

Krieglstein, J. & D. Grusla. 1988. Central depressant constituent in *Valeriana. Deut. Apoth. Zeit.* 128: 2041-6.

Leathwood et al. 1982a. Effect of *Valeriana officinalis* L. on subjective and objective sleep parameters.

Leathwood, P.D. et al. 1982b. Aqueous extract of valerian root *(Valeriana officinalis L.)* improves sleep quality in man.

Pharmacol., Biochem. & Behav. 17: 65-71.

Leung, A. 1980. *Encyclopedia of Common Natural Ingredients Used in Food, Drugs and Cosmetics.* New York: John Wiley & Sons.

Levey, M. 1966. *The Medical Formulary or Aqrabadhin of Al-Kindi.* Madison: The University of Wisconsin Press.

List, P.H. & L. Hörhammer. 1979. *Hagers Handbuch der Pharmazeutischen Praxis.* Berlin: Springer-Verlag.

Long, C. et al. 1989. The chemical constituents of the essential oil from the roots of *Valeriana officinalis* var. *latifolia. Yunan Zhiwu Yanjiu* 9: 109-112.

Lutomski, J. et al. 1975. The effect of drying on the valepotriate content in valerian rhizome. *Herba Polonica* 27: 37-8.

Madaus, G. 1938. *Lehrbuck der Biologischen Heilmittel.* New York: Georg Olms.

Mannenstaetter, E. et al. 1966. Phytochemical studies on *Centranthus ruber. Pharmazie* 21: 321-27.

Marekov, N.L. et al. 1983. Chemistry of pharmaceutically important cyclopentane monoterpenes from some *Valeriana* plants. Chemistry and Biotechnology of Biologically Active Natural Products, 2nd Int. Conf., Budapest, 1983.

Marekov, N.L. et al. Iridoids from Bulgarian Medicinal Plants. *Khim. Ind.* (Sofia) 58: 132-5.

Mary, Z. et al. 1980. Pharmacognostical studies on *Valeriana arnottiana* Wt. and comparison with *V. jatamansi* (=V. wallichii) (Indian valerian). *Herba Hungarica* 19:27-34.

Mathur, J. et al. 1988. In vitro propagation of *Valeriana wallichii. Planta Med.* 54: 82-3.

Medical Societies and Colleges. 1820. *The Pharmacopeia of the United States of America.* Boston: Wells and Lilly.

Milkova, E. et al. 1989. Some aspects of the initiation of callus and suspension cultures of *Valeriana officinalis* var. *Diliana. Acta Biotechnol.* 8: 427-33.

Moore, M. 1979. *Medicinal Plants of the Mountain West.* Santa Fe: Museum of New Mexico Press.

Morvai, M. & I. Molnár-Perl. 1988. Gas Chromatographic Analysis of the Carboxylic Acid Composition of *Valeriana* Extracts. *Chromatographia* 25: 37-42.

Moser, L. 1981. Medicine for stress behind the wheel? *Deutsche Apoth.-Zeit.* 121: 2651-4.

Müller-Limmroth, W. and Ehrenstein. 1977. Untersuchunger über die Wirkungen von Seda-Kneipp auf den Schlaf schlafgestörter Menschen. *Medizinishe Klinik* 72:1119-25.

Ni, M. 1987. *The Tao of Nutrition.* Malibu, CA.: The Shrine of the Eternal Breath of Tao.

Nissen, H.P. et al. 1988. Quality control of plant drugs with HPLC.

GIT Fachz. Lab. 31: 293-5.

Pank, F. et al. 1980. Chemical weed control in the cropping of medicinal plants. *Pharmazie* 35: 115-119.

Parkinson, J. 1640. *Theatrum Botanicum: The Theater of Plants, or An Herball of a Large Extent.* London: Tho. Cotes.

Paxton, J. 1849. *A Pocket Botanical Dictionary.* London: Bradbury & Evans.

Perry, L. 1980. *Medicinal Plants of East and Southeast Asia.* Cambridge, MA: MIT Press.

Pethes, E. & G. Verzár-Petri. 1977. Formation of valepotriates, free low fatty acids and essential oil during ontogeny in the underground part of *Valeriana officinalis* L. *Planta Med.* 30. Pharmazie 41: 499-501.

Petkov, V. & P. Manolov. 1974. To the pharmacology of iridoids. *Chem. Nat. Compds.* 16 B (suppl.): 25-8.

Petkov, V.D. et al. 1973. Pharmacological studies on a mixture of valepotriates isolated from *Valeriana officinalis. Dokl. Bolg. Akad. Nauk* 27: 1007-10. (CA 82: 51636n).

Pickering, C. 1879. *Chronological History of Plants.* Boston: Little, Brown & Co.

Pluta, J. et al. 1981. Investigations of content of heavy metals in chosen dosage forms of drugs of vegetal origin. *Pharmazie* 39: 63.

Popov, S. et al. 1974. A new valepotriate: 7-epi-deacetylisovaltrate from *Valeriana officinalis. Phytochem.* 13: 2815-18.

Pratt, A. [d.m.—ca. 1890]. *The Flowering Plants, Grasses, Sedges, and Ferns of Great Britain.* London: Frederick Warne & Co.

Rashid, M et al. 1973. Active constituents of the rhizomes and roots of *Valeriana officinalis* grown in Egypt in the different seasons of the year and new methods for their determination. *Egypt. J. Pharm. Sci.* 14: 5-11.

Rendle, A.B. 1963. *The Classification of Flowering Plants,* 2 vols. Cambridge: Cambridge University Press.

Renner, A. 1937. The activity of valerians. *Dt. med. Wchschr.* 63: 916-9.

Riedel et al. 1982. Inhibition of GABA breakdown by valerenic acid. *Planta Med.* 46: 219-20.

Roth, L. et al. 1984. *Poisonous Plants—Plant toxins.* Munich: Ecomed.

Roumeliotis, P. & K. K. Unger. 1984. Direct coupling of high-pressure extraction using liquid and supercritical gases to high-pressure liquid chromatography. *Fresenius' Z. Anal. Chem.* 318: 305-6.

Rücker, G. & J. Tautges. 1976. ß-Ionon und patchoulialkohol aus den unterirdischen teilen von *Valeriana officinalis. Phytochem.* 15: 824.

Rücker, G. et al. 1978. Untersuchungen zur Isolierung und pharmakodynamischen Aktivitat des sesquiterpens Valeranion aus *Nardostachys jatamansi* DC. Arzneim-Forsch. 28: 7-13.

Rücker, G. 1979. *Über die Wirkstoffe der Valerianaceen.* Pharmazie in Unserer Zeit 8: 78-86.

Rücker, G. et al. 1982. Quantitative thin-layer chromatographic analysis of valepotriates. *Planta Med.* 43: 299-301.

Rybal'chenko, A.S. et al. 1976. Phenolic compounds of the epigeal part of valerian. *Chem. Nat. Comp.* 12: 98.

Sanyal, D. 1984. *Vegetable Drugs of India.* Dehra Dun: Bishen Singh Mahendra Pal Singh.

Savin, K., et al. 1981. Valerian, *Valeriana officinalis* L., a medicinal plant from some regions of Serbia. *Arh. Farm.* 35: 17-23.

Schätte, R. 1971. Concerning the assay, pharmacology and active constituent formation due to ontological factors of *Radix Valerianae*. Ph.D. Thesis, University of Munich.

Schätte, R. 1972. Stable valerian preparations. *Ger. Offen.* 2,230,626 (Cl. A 61k), 10 Jan 1974. Appl. P 22 30 626.9. (German patents can be ordered through the U.S. patent office). (CA 86: 87504s).

Schellenberg, V. et al. 1993. Quantitative EEG Monitoring in Phyto- and Psycho-Pharmacological Treatment of Psychosomatic and Affective Disorders. *Schizophrenia Research* (2,3).

Shih-Chen, L. 1578. *Pen Ts'ao.* Compiled and translated by Smith, F.P. and G.A. Stuart. San Francisco: Georgetown Press (1973).

Stoll, A. & E. Seebeck. 1958. *1.* Mitt. über Valeriana. Die Isolierung von Hesperitinsäure, Behensäure and zwei unbekannten Säure aus Baldrian. *Rubigs. Ann. Chem.* 603: 158-68.

Stoll, A. et al. 1957. New investigations on Valerian. *Schweizerische Apotheker-Zeitung* 95: 115-120.

Stoll, A. et al. 1958. Isolation and Characterisation of unknown compounds from the neutral fraction of Valerian. *Helv. Chim. Acta.* 40: 1205-30.

Szentpetery, G.R. 1963. Non volatile active principles of Hungarian medicinal valerian. *Pharmazie* 18: 16-18. (CA 60: 10475).

Takamura, K. et al. 1973. Pharmacological actions of *Valeriana officinalis* var. *latifolia. Yakugaku Zasshi* 93: 599-606.

Takamura, K. et al. 1975. Preparations and pharmacological screening of kessoglycol derivatives. *Yakugaku Zasshi* 95: 1198-1209.

Theophrastus. 1948. *Enquiry into Plants,* 2 vols. English Translation by Sir Arthur Hort. Cambridge: Harvard University Press.

Thies, H. 1966. About the constituents of valerian 2: Concerning the constitution of the isovalerianic acid ester valepotriate, acetoxy valepotriate and dihydrovalepotriate. *Tetrahedron Letters:* 11: 1155-62.

Thies, P.W. 1967. Chemistry of the constituents of valepotriate.

Report on the active constituents of Valerian. *Deutsche Apotheker Ztg.* 107: 1411-12.

Thies, P.W. 1968. Active component of valerian. Valerosidatum, an iridoid ester glycoside from *Valeriana* species. *Tetrahedron. Lett.* 28: 2471-4.

Thies, P.W. 1970. Therapeutic isovaleric acid esters. *U.S.* 3,485,857 (ll260,345,C07C) (CA 72: 114873.

Thies, P.W. 1971. Isolation of sedative and spasmolytic isovaleric acid esters from valerian extracts. *Ger. Offen.* 1.617.555 (llA61k) (CA 77: 1972)

Thies, P.W. et al. 1974. On the active agents of Baldrian part 10. The configuration of valtratum and other valepotriates. *Tetrahedron* 29: 3213-26.

Thies, P.W. 1981. About the active constituents of valerians. XIV. Assignment of type and location of the acyloxy substituents in valepotriates via C13-NMR-Spectroscopy. *Planta Med.* 41: 15-20.

Thies, P.W. et al. 1981. Active agents of valerian XIV. assignment of type and location of the acyloxy substituents in valepotriates via carbon-13-NMR spectroscopy. *Planta Med.* 41: 15-20.

Thompson, A.T. 1830. *The London Dispensatory*, 5th ed. London: Longman, Rees, Orme, Brown, and Green.

Thorton, R.J. 1814. *A Family Herbal.* London: R. and R. Crosby and Co.

Tierra, M. 1988. *Planetary Herbology.* Santa Fe: Lotus Press.

Tittel, G. et al. 1978. HPLC-analysis of *Valeriana mexicana* extracts. *Planta Med.* 34: 305-10.

Todd, R.G., ed. 1967. *Extra Pharmacopoeia—Martindale*, 25th ed. London: The Pharmaceutical Press.

Tortarolo, M. et al. 1982. In-vitro effects of epoxide-bearing valepotriates on mouse early hematopoietic progenitor cells and human T-lymphocytes. *Arch. of Toxicol.* 51: 37-42.

Trousseau, A. and H. Pidoux. 1880. *Treatise on Therapeutics*, translated by D.F. Lincoln, 3 vols., 9th ed. New York: William Wood & Co.

Trzhetsinskii, S.D. et al. 1984. Valepotriates of some species of the genus *Valeriana. Chem. Nat. Comp.* 20: 109.

Tutin et al. 1964. *Flora Europa.* Cambridge: Cambridge University Press.

United States Pharmacopeial Convention. 1936. *The Pharmacopeia of the United States of America.* Easton, PA: Mack Printing Co.

Urdang, G. 1944. *Pharmacopoeia Londinensis of 1618* Reproduced in Facsimile With a Historical Introduction. Madison: State Historical Society of Wisconsin.

van Meer, J.H. & R.P. Labadie. 1981. Straight-phase and reversed-phase high-performance liquid chromatographic separations of valepotriate isomers and homologues. *J. of Chromatog.* 205: 206-12.

van Meer, J.H. 1984. Plant constituents with an effect upon the complement system. *Pharmaceutisch Weekblad* 119: 836-42.

Veith et al. 1986. Influence of some breakdown products of valepotriates on the motility of light/dark synchronised mice. *Planta Med.* 179-83.

Vérzarné-Petri, G. 1974. Biosynthesis of alkaloids, valtrates, and volatile oils in the roots of *Valeriana officinalis* from radioactive precursors. *Acta. Pharm. Hung.* 44, Suppl. 54-65.

Vérzarné-Petri, G. et al. 1977. Thin-layer and gas chromatographic studies on iridoid compounds in *Valeriana officinalis* L. *Herba Hung.* 15: 79-91

Violon, C. et al. 1983. Microscopical study of valepotriates in lipid droplets of various tissues from valerian plants. *Plant Cell Reports* 2: 300-3.

Violon, C. 1984. Relation between valepotriate content and differentiation level in various tissues from *Valerianaceae. J. of Nat. Prod.* 47: 934-40.

Violon, C. et al. 1984. Comparative study of the essential oils of in vivo and in vitro grown *Valeriana officinalis* L. and *Centranthus macrosiphon Boiss.* by coupled gas chromatograpy-mass spectrometry. *J. of Chromatog.* 288: 474-78.

Voigt, S. et al. 1978. Biosynthesis and metabolism of constituents with an epoxide structure. *Pharmazie* 33: 632.

von Eickstedt, K.-W. & S. Rahman. 1969. Psychopharmacologic effects of the valepotriates. *Arzneim.-Forsch.* 19: 316-19.

von Eickstedt, K.-W. 1969. Influence on the effects of alcohol by the valepotriates. *Arzneim.-Forsch.* 19: 995-7.

Wagner, H. & K. Jurcic. 1979. About the spasmolytic effects of valerians. *Planta Med.* 37: 84-6.

Wagner, H. 1972. On the dependence of the valepotriate and ethereal oil content in *Valerian officinalis* L.s.l. upon different exogenous and endogenous factors. *Arznei.-Forsch.* 22: 1204-9.

Wagner, H. 1980. Comparative studies on the sedative action of *Valeriana* extracts, valepotriates and their degradation products. *Planta Med.* 38: 358-65.

Wagner, H. 1984. *Plant Drug Analysis* (English ed.). New York: Springer-Verlag.

Wagner, H., & P. Wolff. 1977. *New Natural Products and Plant Drugs with Pharmacological, Biological or Therapeutical Activity.* New York: Springer-Verlag.

Walker, W. 1958. *All the Plants of the Bible.* London: Lutterworth Press.

Wallis, T.E. 1955. *Textbook of Pharmacognosy.* London: J. & A. Churchill.

Wang, Z.-Y. & F.-D. Niu. 1980. Studies on the chemical constituents of the essential oil of *Valeriana jatamansi* Jones., Yun-nan Chih Wu Yen Chiu 2: 58-61.

Weiss, R.F. 1988. *Herbal Medicine.* Beaconsfield, England: Beaconsfield Publishers Ltd.

Wichtl, M. 1978. Drug analysis and pharmacopeias, a critical survey. *Planta Med.* 34: 113-28.

Wienschierz, H.-J. 1978. Experience with cultivation of *Valeriana wallichii* D.C. in the Federal Republic of German. *Acta Hort.* 73: 315-329.

Wilson, C.O. et al. (eds.). 1977. *Textbook of Organic and Pharmaceutical Chemistry.* Philadelphia: J.B. Lippincott.

Woodville, W. 1790. *Medical Botany,* 3 vols. London: James Phillips (for the author).

Youngken, H.W. 1950. *Textbook of Pharmacognosy,* 6th ed. Philadelphia: The Blakiston Co.

Zeylstra, H. 1984. *Valerian, a Review.* National Institute of Medical Herbalists. Tunbridge Wells, England.